# PEDIATRIC COLLECTIONS
# Pulmonology Cases

**EDITED BY:**

**Catherine Kier, MD, MHA, FAAP**
Professor of Clinical Pediatrics and Division Chief, Pediatric Pulmonary
Stony Brook Children's Hospital
Renaissance School of Medicine, Stony Brook University

# American Academy of Pediatrics
## DEDICATED TO THE HEALTH OF ALL CHILDREN®

**Published by the American Academy of Pediatrics**
**345 Park Blvd.**
**Itasca, IL 60143**

APC047

Print ISBN: 978-1-61002-816-5
eBook ISBN: 978-1-61002-817-2

# PEDIATRIC COLLECTIONS
# Pulmonology Cases

## Table of Contents

**Pulmonology Cases: Case Reports from *Pediatrics in Review***

## About AAP Pediatric Collections

Pediatric Collections is a series of selected pediatric articles that highlight different facets of information across various AAP publications, including AAP Journals, AAP News, Blog Articles, and eBooks. Each series of collections focuses on specific topics in the field of pediatrics so that you can keep up with best practices and make an informed response to public health matters, trending news, and current events. Each collection includes previously published content focusing on specific topics and articles selected by AAP editors.

Visit http://collections.aap.org to view current online collections.

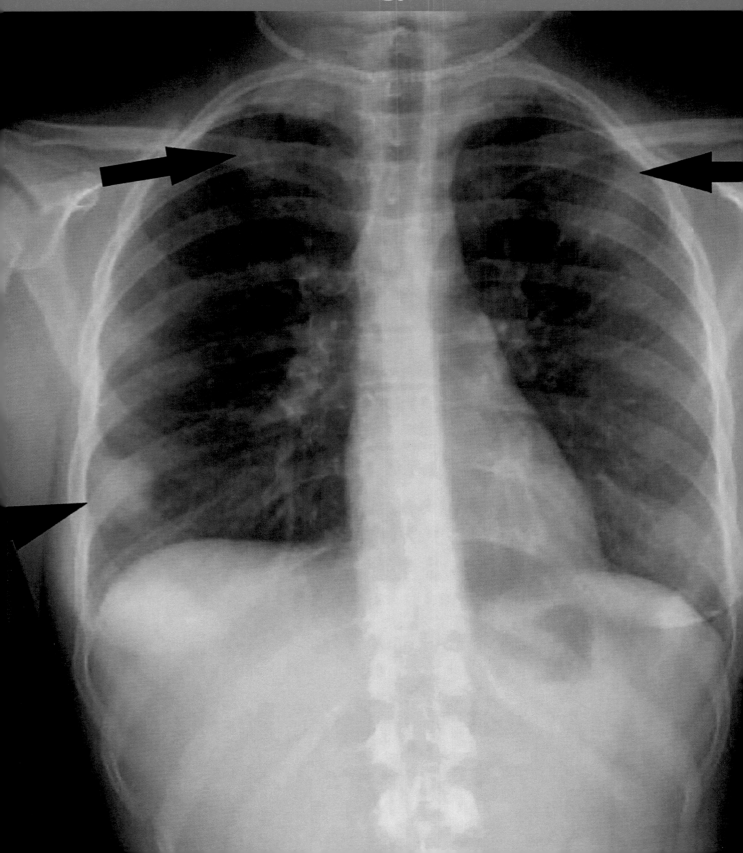

# Pulmonology Cases
## Collection Introduction

**Catherine Kier, MD, MHA, FAAP**
Professor of Clinical Pediatrics and Division Chief, Pediatric Pulmonary
Stony Brook Children's Hospital
Renaissance School of Medicine, Stony Brook University

The articles in this compilation of respiratory-related clinical cases remind us that the field of pediatric pulmonology encompasses everything from the upper airway to the lower airway to the pulmonary manifestations of a systemic disease. As clinicians we must be aware of the different causes of hypoxemia and the differential diagnosis of a cough as well as approach respiratory distress with a slew of possible diagnoses, congenital abnormalities, and, of course, what we may have learned new from the recent COVID-19 pandemic. Knowing the patho-physiology of diseases is key to the critical thinking that leads to the best possible diagnosis. This review of cases reminds us that it is the journey that teaches the learner how to arrive at the correct diagnosis.

Case-based learning as a teaching method in medical education makes learners develop critical thinking and clinical reasoning skills. Being actively engaged in the learning process makes one become inquisitive and become more comfortable in carving the path to an eventual diagnosis.

It brings me back to my medical school and residency days, remembering the phrase of Theodore Woodward, MD (1914–2005), an excellent medical educator: "When you hear hoofbeats, think horses, not zebras." Indeed, respiratory distress in a young child or infant who is other-wise healthy, amid respiratory viral season, likely has bronchiolitis. Asthma is the most common chronic respiratory illness in childhood, and if there is a high predictive index (such as history of asthma in one or both parents, evidence of atopy, eczema, rhinitis, high blood eosinophil count, or presence of aeroallergens), then we have used one of the many things in our toolbox, as clinicians, and could reserve further work-up only in otherwise puzzling cases or cases that do not quite fit the usual diagnosis. Most diagnoses are common (horses), but there are a few that challenge us, and there is a chance that some may be a rare diagnosis (zebra). Autoimmune, immunodeficiency, and eosinophilic diseases may be "zebras" of asthma at times.

It is good clinical practice to always review information carefully as we gather it from history and from physical exam. We draw information especially from what strikes us the moment we walk in the exam room or at bedside, such as noisy breathing or stridor, for example. Ordering a test, whether it is blood work or imaging (such as chest radiography or computed tomography scans of the chest), should always be thoughtful and not routine, asking the question of how the information will help in producing a diagnosis or getting closer to an answer. Medical literature is so rich with cases and guidance that it is best practice to peruse respected websites and online libraries to aid in one's decision-making. By making it a consistent practice to check and read the literature as interesting clinical cases come up, one's knowledge base gets richer. Medical advances are at such a fast pace that keeping up and asking the expert will keep us on track. Cystic fibrosis (CF) as a disease, for example, may present very differently from the typical clinical presentation just a decade or two ago. The predicted median survival (among people with CF born 2019–2023), is beyond 60 years of age based on the most recent CF regis-try (2023), CF newborn screening is universal across all 50 states, and many disease-causing variants (formerly known as mutations) are now detected through comprehensive genetic testing. This leads to a more diverse CF population each year. Additionally, the availability of the highly effective modulator therapy significantly changed the trajectory of the disease. Yet, we must know our basics and foundation for the disease. Finding a nasal polyp on a teenager who cannot smell (anosmia) but who has a history of pancreatitis as well should lead one to order a sweat test to rule out CF.

The standard format for the Index of Suspicion, used consistently, makes the compilation of the subspecialty cases an effective way of teaching learners to formulate strategies for their "detective" skills. As a medical educator, I find these cases extremely helpful in facilitating learning, by suggesting ways for learners to improve their clinical reasoning skills and to improve their presentations. Supporting them during discussion of uncertainties in diagnoses will make them more comfortable and thus more engaged in active learning.

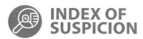

# INDEX OF SUSPICION

# Anemia and a New Supplemental Oxygen Requirement in a 2-year-old Boy

Olivia Crowe, MD,[§] RosaMarie Maiorella, MD,[*†] Aki Tanimoto, MD,[†‡] Shivani J. Patel, DO, MEd, MS[*†]

[*]Division of Hospital Medicine, Cincinnati Children's Hospital Medical Center, Cincinnati, OH
[†]Department of Pediatrics, University of Cincinnati, College of Medicine, Cincinnati, OH
[‡]Department of Radiology, Cincinnati Children's Hospital Medical Center, Cincinnati, OH
[§]Department of Pediatrics, University of Cincinnati, and Cincinnati Children's Hospital, Cincinnati, OH

## PRESENTATION

A 22-month-old unimmunized boy born at 27 weeks and 5 days with a history of bronchopulmonary dysplasia, now resolved; patent ductus arteriosus status postclosure by an occlusion device; and pulmonary hypertension with mild right systolic dysfunction presents to the emergency department (ED) with 3 weeks of worsening fatigue and 1 day of pallor. He eats a good balance of fruits, vegetables, and protein but drinks 74 oz of almond milk daily. On review of his growth chart, he has persistently been at less than the fifth percentile for both weight and length but has been following his curve. His family history is remarkable for maternal systemic lupus erythematosus (SLE). He has not received any of his vaccines because of maternal religious beliefs.

In the ED, he is well-appearing although pale, with vital signs significant for a temperature of 100.8 °F (38.22°C), heart rate of 162 beats/min, respiratory rate of 28 breaths/min, and oxygen saturation (Spo$_2$) of 85%. On examination, heart sounds are notable for tachycardia without a murmur, lungs are clear to auscultation bilaterally, and he has no increased work of breathing apart from tachypnea. He is placed on a 2-L nasal cannula with improvement in his Spo$_2$ to the high 90s. Initial laboratory results reveal a hemoglobin of 2.7 gm/dL (decreased from 10.7 gm/dL 3 months before), mean corpuscular volume of 66.3 fL, and normal total bilirubin. A chest radiograph reveals bilateral opacities and is read as a potential community-acquired pneumonia (CAP) (Fig 1A). He is started on ampicillin and admitted to hospital medicine for further patient management.

On the acute care unit, hematology is consulted. Iron studies reveal an elevated total iron-binding capacity at 469 μg/dL and a low percentage of saturation at 2%. His absolute reticulocyte count is not elevated despite his anemia. He receives a total of 20 cc/kg of packed red blood cells over 2 days with an increase in his hemoglobin to 7.1 gm/dL. He also receives 300 mg of iron infusions for potential iron deficiency anemia and completes a 7-day course of amoxicillin for CAP. A repeat chest radiograph is obtained after he has a persistent oxygen requirement, and this reveals increasing bilateral opacities with confluent opacities at the lung bases, concerning for fluid overload (Fig 1B). With his history of right-sided systolic dysfunction, an echocardiogram is obtained, which reveals that his heart function has normalized. He is given furosemide with a subsequent decrease in his oxygen requirement but remains unable to wean to room air. A repeat complete blood cell count is then obtained and is notable for a decrease in his hemoglobin from 7.1 gm/dL to

AUTHOR DISCLOSURE: Drs Crowe, Maiorella, Tanimoto, and Patel have disclosed no financial relationships relevant to this article. This commentary does not contain a discussion of an unapproved/investigative use of a commercial product/device.

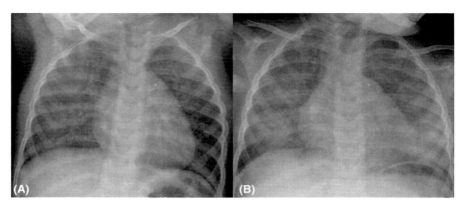

**Figure 1.** A. Frontal chest radiograph reveals patchy opacities throughout the right lung and patchy left apical opacities. B. Frontal chest radiograph after red blood cell transfusion and iron infusion reveals increased basilar predominant patchy and confluent opacities. Differential considerations in this setting include increased permeability edema secondary to transfusion, edema from volume overload, worsening infection, diffuse alveolar damage, as well as DAH. DAH=diffuse alveolar hemorrhage.

6 gm/dL. This prompts a reevaluation of the presumed diagnosis of iron deficiency anemia and initiation of a further evaluation.

## DISCUSSION

### Differential Diagnosis

The patient's persistent oxygen requirement and acute decrease in hemoglobin after transfusion was inconsistent with the initial diagnosis of iron deficiency anemia and CAP. Anemia itself does not cause a decrease in oxygen saturation measured via pulse oximetry ($spo_2$) because available hemoglobin still binds to oxygen. Therefore, we needed to consider other diseases that could explain both these findings, namely those causing hemolysis or hemorrhage. A laboratory evaluation for hemolytic anemia was remarkable for an elevated lactate dehydrogenase at 952 U/L, a low haptoglobin at less than 8 mg/dL, and elevated total bilirubin at 3.4 mg/dL. Given the maternal history of SLE, autoimmune hemolytic anemias were considered but were less likely after a direct antiglobulin test antibody test results and direct antiglobulin test-negative hemolytic anemia panel results were both negative. In terms of possible sites of hemorrhage, a fecal occult blood test was obtained to assess for gastrointestinal bleeding and yielded a negative result. An ultrasonography of the liver and spleen was negative for hematoma. A computed tomography pulmonary angiogram was then obtained to evaluate pulmonary etiologies and revealed diffuse parenchymal opacities with a gravity-dependent gradient (Fig 2). Although this is a nonspecific finding, it is concerning for pulmonary hemorrhage.

Diffuse alveolar hemorrhage (DAH) can be caused by a broad array of diseases with or without pulmonary capillaritis. (1) A hallmark feature for all causes of DAH is finding hemosiderin-laden macrophages in samples collected by bronchoalveolar lavage (BAL) because macrophages are responsible for clearing the erythrocytes from the alveoli. (1) In this case, we initially considered autoimmune processes leading to DAH via vasculitis (anti-glomerular basement membrane syndrome (Goodpasture syndrome), granulomatosis with polyangiitis (formerly Wegener Granulomatosis, etc), but the result of a rheumatologic evaluation, including antinuclear antibody, antineutrophilic cytoplasmic antibody profile, and anti-double stranded DNA, was negative, and a urinalysis was normal without hematuria. Cardiovascular etiologies, such as pulmonary hypertension, were unlikely with a normal echocardiogram. Another cause of DAH is idiopathic pulmonary hemosiderosis (IPH), a diagnosis of exclusion. After a multidisciplinary discussion with hospital medicine, hematology, and pulmonology, the family agreed to proceed with bronchoscopy with bronchoalveolar lavage (BAL). The BAL revealed signs of acute-on-chronic pulmonary hemorrhage with 80% of macrophages containing coarse hemosiderin. Bacterial and fungal cultures were obtained and had no growth. The findings on the BAL, in combination with an otherwise negative-result evaluation, confirmed the diagnosis of IPH.

### The Condition

IPH is a rare condition, the pathogenesis of which is still largely unknown. It is characterized by recurrent episodes of DAH without a known cause. In one single-center study, IPH was found to be the most common cause of DAH in pediatric individuals, accounting for 65% of cases over 10 years. (2) Its incidence ranges between 0.24 and 1.23 children per million on the basis of the population. (3)(4) There is likely an immunologic association because many individuals will have intermittent autoantibody seropositivity, and most improve

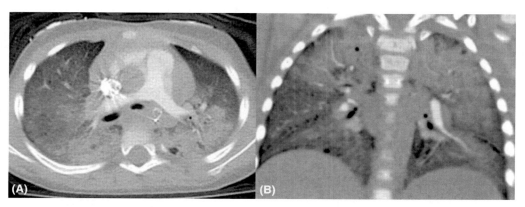

**Figure 2.** A. Axial image from chest CT scan reveals bilateral ground-glass opacities with dependent consolidation. B. Coronal image highlights apical predominance of findings, likely secondary to recumbent positioning. CT scan findings are suggestive of diffuse alveolar damage, DAH, atypical infection, and less likely edema given the lack of pleural effusions and interlobular septal thickening. CT=computed tomography; DAH=diffuse alveolar hemorrhage.

with immunosuppressive therapy. (5) In addition, IPH can cooccur with celiac disease, also known as Lane-Hamilton syndrome. (6)(7) Consideration has also been given to a genetic component because the prevalence in pediatric individuals who have Down syndrome is up to 75 times higher, although a specific gene locus has not been identified. (4) Other possible risk factors include environmental exposures, such as to secondhand smoke or indoor mold. (3)(6)

The classic triad for IPH (hemoptysis, iron deficiency anemia, and pulmonary infiltrates on chest radiograph) is not always seen in children. (3) In one study, a quarter of children presented with anemia as their only symptom; this may account for a high rate of misdiagnosis at initial presentation. (3) Other common presenting symptoms include cough, hemoptysis, and dyspnea. (3)(4) Patients can develop a supplemental oxygen requirement as the degree of hemorrhage worsens and more areas of the lungs are involved. Initial evaluation begins with a chest radiograph, which can reveal either diffuse alveolar opacities or an interstitial pattern depending on the length of time since hemorrhage last occurred. (6) Chest computed tomography (CT) scan provides greater sensitivity than chest radiographs for parenchymal abnormality and may reveal findings of hemorrhage, including ground-glass opacities and consolidation. (6) The gold standard for diagnosis is lung biopsy; however, this is rarely performed in children because of its invasive nature. (3)(6) Instead, sputum, gastric fluid, or BAL samples can be examined for hemosiderin-laden macrophages with sensitivities of 92%, 98%, and 100%, respectively. (3) BAL with cultures is recommended to rule out potential infection. (6)

Systemic corticosteroids are the first-line choice for both induction and maintenance therapy. In pediatric individuals, clinicians often use oral prednisone at a dose of 2 mg/kg per day for induction. (5) In cases of life-threatening hemorrhage causing acute respiratory failure, treatment may start with pulse steroids at doses of 10 to 30 mg/kg per day for 3 days. (3)(5)(8) The induction dose can then be tapered to a maintenance dose after 4 to 8 weeks if there are no recurrent episodes. (5) Maintenance therapy is continued for 12 to 18 months, after which steroids may be tapered and discontinued if symptoms have not returned. (5) Importantly, there are no evidence-based guidelines on the initial dosing of systemic corticosteroid therapy because of the lack of randomized control trials; current dosing is solely dependent on case reports. (8) Recurrence is common, particularly in children. Risk factors for recurrence include hypoxia and the requirement of blood transfusion at diagnosis. (9) In one study, children who suffered from recurrent hemorrhage had an average of 3.6 episodes each with a median recurrence time of 6 months after cessation of steroids (9).

## Patient Course

After the bronchoscopy, the patient was transferred to the pulmonology service, in which he completed a 3-day course of pulse steroids at 10 mg/kg per day. He was then transitioned to daily steroids of 2 mg/kg. He was able to wean to room air during the day with supplemental oxygen at night. He was discharged from the hospital with plans to follow up with pulmonology as well as his clinician for further discussion regarding immunizations given his immunosuppressed status. However, the patient had multiple risk factors for recurrence (hypoxia, blood transfusion at time of diagnosis) and represented to the hospital a few weeks later with a recurrent episode requiring re-initiation of pulse steroids.

Lessons for the Clinician

- Anemia itself does not cause a decrease in oxygen saturation. The clinician should consider other causes if patients have a persistent supplemental oxygen requirement.
- The classic triad of hemoptysis, iron deficiency anemia, and pulmonary infiltrates is rarely seen in children with IPH. Many children present with only anemia and no pulmonary symptoms.
- BAL is recommended for diagnosis to visualize hemosiderin-laden macrophages and rule out infection.
- Steroids are initiated at higher doses to induce remission and then are slowly tapered to a maintenance dose, which may be discontinued in 12 to 18 months if symptoms do not recur.

*References for this article can be found at*
*https://doi.org/10.1542/pir.2022-005663*

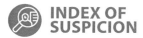 **INDEX OF SUSPICION**

# Cyanosis in a Previously Well Child

Moodakare A. Bhat, MBBS,[*] Matthew R. Plunk, MD,[‡] Donald G. Basel, MD,[†] Sheila J. Hanson, MD, MS[*]

[*]Division of Critical Care and
[†]Division of Medical Genetics, Department of Pediatrics, and
[‡]Division of Pediatric Radiology, Department of Radiology, Medical College of Wisconsin, Milwaukee, WI

## PRESENTATION

A previously healthy 12-year-old boy is seen for a health supervision visit by his pediatrician. Clinical examination is significant for cyanosis of his lips, mucus membranes, and hands, and clubbing of fingers. He has not seen a primary care provider in the past 3 years. He is able to play, bike, be involved in physical education activities in school, and keep up with peers in physical activities without shortness of breath or fatigue. He reports self-limiting episodes of epistaxis once or twice a year for the past 2 to 3 years. He has not traveled outside the country. Family history is unrevealing. Pulse oximetry shows oxygen saturation of 75% to 80%. His heart rate is 70 beats/min, respiratory rate is 20 breaths/min, and blood pressure is 100/52 mm Hg in the right arm in a sitting position, with no difference in blood pressure between the upper and lower extremities. His weight is 41 kg (36th percentile for age) and height is 149 cm (33rd percentile for age). Respiratory and cardiac examination findings are normal. He is referred to a local emergency department for further management of severe hypoxemia. In the emergency department he has no improvement in oxygen saturation with oxygen therapy. A capillary blood gas analysis shows oxygen saturation of 79% (reference range, 90%–100%), with arterial partial pressure of oxygen ($Pao_2$) of 40 mm Hg (reference range, 60–80 mm Hg) and partial pressure of carbon dioxide of 35 mm Hg (reference range, 35–35 mm Hg). Blood methemoglobin level is undetectable. Electrolyte levels are normal. Complete blood count is significant for a hemoglobin (Hb) level of 20 g/dL (200 g/L) (reference range, 12–16 g/dL [120–160 g/L]) and a hematocrit value of 59% (reference range, 36%–47%). An echocardiogram, performed without a bubble study, shows no structural abnormalities and normal cardiac function. A chest radiograph shows focal opacity of the left upper lobe. A chest computed tomographic scan reveals the diagnosis.

## DISCUSSION

### Differential Diagnosis

It is important to differentiate between hypoxemia (decreased $Pao_2$ in the blood) and hypoxia (decreased tissue oxygenation).

Oxygen content of blood is dependent on Hb and the degree of saturation with oxygen, which in turn is dependent on the partial pressure of oxygen in the blood: oxygen content of blood (mL/dL) = 1.36 × Hb (g/dL) × oxygen saturation / 100 + 0.003 × $Pao_2$ (mm Hg).

**AUTHOR DISCLOSURE** Drs Bhat, Plunk, Basel, and Hanson have disclosed no financial relationships relevant to this article. This commentary does not contain a discussion of an unapproved/investigative use of a commercial product/device.

Patients can compensate for chronic hypoxemia by increasing blood Hb concentrations, thereby increasing the oxygen content of the blood to maintain adequate tissue-level oxygenation. During acute hypoxemia, the body is unable to compensate, and hypoxia often ensues.

Conversely, the tissues maybe unable to obtain adequate oxygen, despite normal $Pao_2$, due to conditions affecting either the quality (carbon monoxide poisoning, methemoglobinemia) or quantity (anemia) of Hb.

Hypoxemia could be secondary to hypoventilation, diffusion limitation of oxygen at the alveolar capillary membrane, or ventilation-perfusion mismatch (ie, inadequate perfusion of ventilated parts of the lung) or due to a right-to-left shunt (Table 1). Hypoxemia due to all these causes except a shunt lesion is responsive to supplemental oxygen. (1) Shunt lesions could be secondary to intrapulmonary shunt or due to an intracardiac shunt.

Rarely, uncorrected cyanotic heart disease can present similarly. By adolescence, patients have growth restriction, poor exercise tolerance, and polycythemia and can have a poor prognosis. They are at risk for complications secondary to polycythemia and paradoxical embolism such as strokes and brain abscesses. Usually emboli in the systemic circulation are derived from thrombi in the ventricle. However, in the presence of an intracardiac or intrapulmonary shunt, an embolus from a thrombus in the venous side can cross over to the arterial side, causing embolism in the systemic circulation. This is known as paradoxical embolism. (2) Tetralogy of Fallot and Ebstein anomaly are the most common cyanotic lesions presenting in later childhood. Tetralogy of Fallot is characterized by a large ventricular septal defect, an aorta that overrides the left and right ventricles, obstruction of the right ventricular outflow tract, and right ventricular hypertrophy. The degree of cyanosis depends on the degree of obstruction to the right ventricular outflow tract. Mild obstruction is initially well tolerated, but symptoms usually develop by adolescence. In Ebstein anomaly, displacement of posterior and septal leaflets of the tricuspid valves into the right ventricle results in atrialization of a variable amount of right ventricular myocardium. This results in a variable degree of tricuspid regurgitation, leading to development of right-sided heart failure and cyanosis due to increased right atrial pressures and development of a right-to-left shunt in the presence of a patent foramen ovale. If the degree of displacement is not severe, patients may initially remain asymptomatic. Ebstein anomaly is associated with atrial tachycardias and atrioventricular nodal reentrant tachycardias. Adults and adolescents often come to medical attention due to symptoms of these arrhythmias. (3) In Eisenmenger syndrome, a large long-standing left-to-right intracardiac shunt such as a ventricular septal defect or patent ductus arteriosus causes severe pulmonary vascular disease and pulmonary hypertension, with resultant reversal of the direction of shunting and development of cyanosis. (4)

Methemoglobin is an altered form of Hb where the iron is present in its oxidized ferric form instead of in the normal ferrous form. Methemoglobin is unable to bind to oxygen. Methemoglobin also causes left shift of the oxyhemoglobin curve, decreasing release of oxygen from normal oxyhemoglobin to the tissues. In methemoglobinemia, only transport of oxygen by Hb is altered, but $Pao_2$ in the blood is normal. Thus, in methemoglobinemia, although oxygen saturation measured by pulse oximetry is low, $Pao_2$ on blood gas is normal. These mechanisms result in tissue hypoxia without hypoxemia. Methemoglobinemia is usually caused by exposure to substances that cause oxidation of iron, such as topical anesthetics (benzocaine and prilocaine) and water with high nitrate content (some well

**Table 1.** Causes of Hypoxemia

| MECHANISM | RESPONSE TO SUPPLEMENTAL OXYGEN | EXAMPLES |
|---|---|---|
| Hypoventilation | Yes | Central hypoventilation, opioid overdose |
| Diffusion limitation: Oxygen is unable to diffuse across the alveolocapillary membrane | Yes | Lung disease: interstitial lung disease, emphysema |
| Ventilation-perfusion mismatch: Areas of the lung have high perfusion without adequate ventilation; leads to build up of $CO_2$ and secondary drop in oxygen concentration in those areas | Yes | Atelectasis, acute respiratory distress syndrome |
| Shunt lesion: Proportion of total blood flow bypasses the lung and does not take part in gas exchange | No | Intracardiac shunt: cyanotic heart diseases Intrapulmonary shunt: arteriovenous malformations |

water). Congenital forms of methemoglobinemia secondary to cytochrome b5 reductase deficiency, cytochrome b5 deficiency, or Hb M disease also occur. These forms present with mildly decreased oxygen saturation on pulse oximetry at birth. Hypoxia can be exacerbated by exposure to oxidizing substances. (5)

Pulmonary arteriovenous malformations (PAVMs) associated with hereditary hemorrhagic telangiectasia (HHT) 90% of the time can occasionally be idiopathic. They can also occur secondary to infections such as schistosomiasis and actinomycosis, trauma, hepatopulmonary syndrome, and cavopulmonary shunts. Cavopulmonary shunts, such as the Glenn and Fontan shunts, connecting inferior and superior vena cava, respectively, to the pulmonary artery, are surgically created to palliate cardiac lesions with single ventricle physiology. Hepatopulmonary syndrome is thought to result from abnormal vasodilatory metabolites that are not metabolized owing to liver failure entering the lung. They cause microscopic vascular dilatations in the lung. This results in symptoms of an intrapulmonary shunt of hypoxemia and orthodeoxia. (6)(7)(8) Abernethy malformation is a rare cause of PAVM. It is characterized by the persistence of embryonic vessels, resulting in a direct communication between the portal and systemic venous circulations. It is associated with Down syndrome, Turner syndrome, and congenital cardiac disease. Clinical presentation can range from asymptomatic to hepatopulmonary syndrome, encephalopathy secondary to hyperammonemia, and pulmonary hypertension. (7)

Capillary malformation AVM (CM-AVM) syndrome, a genetic disorder causing a variety of AVMs, is caused by mutation of the RASA-1 gene and does not result in hypoxemia.

## Actual Diagnosis

Multiple PAVMs were present throughout both lungs. A dominant AVM large enough to account for the opacity on the chest radiograph was present in the posterior portion of the left upper lobe, and numerous smaller AVMs were present throughout the lung (Fig). Based on clinical findings of PAVMs and epistaxis, a diagnosis of possible HHT was made, and the patient underwent genetic testing for HHT. The HHT gene panel identified a pathogenic variant in the ENG gene, confirming the diagnosis. He underwent digital subtraction pulmonary angiography with staged embolization of PAVMs. A complex AVM was present in the left upper lobe with at least 3 dominant arterial feeders. Two more prominent malformations were located in the right middle lobe and the right lower lobe. Numerous smaller

AVMs were present throughout the lung. After the procedures his oxygen saturation improved to 90% to 92%, with presence of residual shunting in the smaller AVMs. He continues to be managed by a multidisciplinary team of pulmonologists, geneticists, and radiologists.

## The Condition

HHT (or Osler-Weber-Rendu disease) is an autosomal dominant disorder characterized by AVMs predominantly in the lungs, liver, brain, gastrointestinal tract, and mucocutaneous telangiectasias. Diagnosis is based on the Curaçao criteria (Table 2) and confirmed by genetic testing for pathogenic variants in the ENG, ACVRL1, SMAD4, GDF2, and BMP9 genes. ENG and ACVRL1 gene variations account for 85% of cases. The SMAD4 mutation increases the risk of juvenile polyposis. (9) HHT exhibits age-related penetrance, with almost all affected individuals exhibiting symptoms by age 40 years. Although visceral AVMs are mostly congenital, new visceral AVMs can develop over time in HHT. (9)(10)

Epistaxis is the most common clinical symptom, developing in approximately 50% of patients by age 10 years and in 85% to 90% by age 20 years. Severe epistaxis, typically described as nosebleeds unresponsive to local pressure, is common with truncating pathogenic variants involving ACVRL1. (11)

PAVMs are present in 30% to 60% of patients with HHT. PAVMs tend to increase in size over time. PAVMs consist of 1 or more feeding arteries, an aneurysmal sac, and 1 or more draining veins, without an intervening capillary bed. Most feeding arteries arise from the pulmonary arteries, and draining veins drain into branches of the pulmonary vein. Diffuse PAVMs involve multiple subsegmental arteries and have poorer prognosis and higher rates of complications. (12)

PAVMs result in right-to-left shunting, leading to significant hypoxemia. PAVMs are most frequent in the lower lobes of the lungs, which can cause orthodeoxia (desaturation when the patient is upright) due to preferential redistribution of blood into the PAVMs in the upright position. Rarely, the aneurysmal sac wall can rupture, causing massive hemoptysis. Right-to-left shunting can also lead to strokes and brain abscesses. Rarely, PAVM rupture into the pleural space can lead to air embolism. Pulmonary hypertension secondary to hypoxic vasoconstriction can develop over time.

Transthoracic contrast echocardiography is the recommended screening tool. Transthoracic contrast echocardiography with agitated saline, also known as a bubble

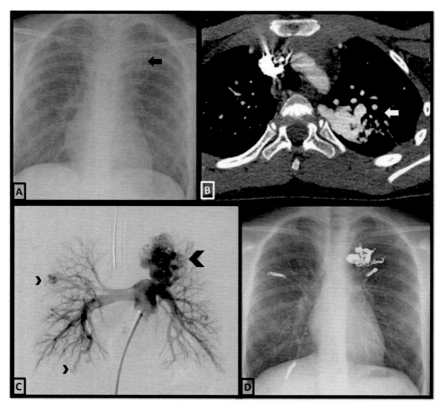

**Figure.** Pulmonary arteriovenous malformations (AVMs) on imaging. A. Initial chest radiograph with left upper lobe opacity (black arrow). B. Contrast-enhanced computed tomographic scan shows a large, complex AVM in the left upper lobe (white arrow). C. Digital subtraction pulmonary angiogram from the main pulmonary artery with a dominant AVM (arrowhead) and additional AVMs in the right lung (smaller arrowheads). D. Postembolization chest radiograph showing multiple coils used for embolotherapy.

study, has 99% to 100% sensitivity. Agitated saline with air bubbles is injected through a peripheral intravenous catheter. Visualization of air bubbles in the left side of the heart after 3 to 4 cardiac cycles is suggestive of an intrapulmonary shunt, whereas visualization within 1 to 2 seconds is suggestive of an intracardiac shunt. (13)

Chest computed tomography is the gold standard; contrast injection is typically unnecessary for visualization of

these lesions. Magnetic resonance angiography can also be helpful, especially in planning for intervention and avoidance of radiation exposure.

The decision to intervene on PAVMs is based on multiple factors, including size of feeding arteries. Intervention is recommended for PAVMs with feeder arteries greater than 3 mm. Other factors that influence decision making to intervene on PAVMs with smaller feeder arteries

**Table 2.** Curaçao Criteria for Clinical Diagnosis of HHT

Spontaneous and recurrent epistaxis
Multiple telangiectasias at characteristic sites: lips, oral cavity, fingers, nose
Visceral lesions: gastrointestinal telangiectasia, pulmonary, hepatic, cerebral, or spinal arteriovenous malformations
A first-degree relative with HHT
Definitive diagnosis ≥3 criteria are present
   Possible or suspected diagnosis 2 criteria are present
      Unlikely diagnosis <2 criteria are present[a]

HHT=hereditary hemorrhagic telangiectasia.
[a]According to experts in the 2011 HHT Guidelines Working Group, identifying fewer than 2 criteria should not be sufficient to rule out the diagnosis of HHT because signs are not always apparent in the first few decades of life. (15)
Adapted from Shovlin CL, Guttmacher AE, Buscarini E, et al. Diagnostic criteria for hereditary hemorrhagic telangiectasia (Rendu-Osler-Weber syndrome). *Am J Med Genet.* 2000;91(1):66–67. (8)

include presence of and perceived risk of neurologic complications and pulmonary hemorrhage, exercise limitations of the patient, and technical challenges of the procedure. Percutaneous image-guided embolotherapy is currently the treatment of choice. Diffuse type of PAVMs can involve an entire segment of the lung and are harder to manage and can require surgical intervention or, rarely, lung transplant. (10)(13)(14)

In the absence of PAVMs, if HHT is suspected based on Curaçao criteria, and is confirmed by genetic testing, screening for PAVMs should be undertaken at the time of diagnosis of HHT. If negative, rescreening is recommended at puberty, within 5 years of a planned pregnancy, after a pregnancy, and every 5 to 10 years. Antibiotic prophylaxis for procedures with risk of bacteremia is recommended. Avoidance of scuba diving is also recommended due to a theoretical increased risk of cerebral embolism from decompression and paradoxical embolism through the PAVM. Extra care must be taken to avoid air embolism when any intravenous access is placed. (15)

Cerebrovascular malformations, including cerebral AVMs, micro AVMs (<1 cm in size), AV fistulas, and telangiectasias, are present in 11% to 16% of patients with HHT. Screening for cerebrovascular malformations for all patients with HHT using brain MRI is recommended. (15)

Screening for gastrointestinal AVMs is recommended only in symptomatic patients and in patients with juvenile polyposis/HHT subtype because gastrointestinal AVMs in the former subtypes are usually asymptomatic. When symptomatic, they present as iron deficiency anemia, secondary to chronic gastrointestinal bleeding. Screening for liver AVMs with Doppler ultrasonography should be considered in patients with elevated liver enzyme levels, symptoms of portal hypertension, biliary or intestinal ischemia, or high-output heart failure. (15)

## Lessons for the Clinician

- Pulmonary arteriovenous malformations (PAVMs) can present with varying degrees of cyanosis in an asymptomatic child. Hypoxemia in PAVM is not responsive to oxygen. Orthodeoxia, or increase in hypoxemia with upright position, is another sign suggestive of PAVM.
- Hereditary hemorrhagic telangiectasia (HHT) is characterized by AVMs involving multiple organs resulting in a variety of complications. Early diagnosis and treatment of PAVMs and cerebral AVMs are crucial due to serious consequences of rupture of a cerebral AVM and paradoxical embolism from a PAVM.
- Greater than 90% of spontaneous PAVMs are associated with HHT, and diagnosis is based on Curaçao criteria and genetic testing for HHT.
- Patients with PAVMs are at risk for paradoxical embolism, and antibiotic prophylaxis is recommended for patients undergoing procedures at risk for septic embolization. These patients must avoid scuba diving.
- Hypoxemia could be secondary to hypoventilation, diffusion limitation of oxygen at the alveolar capillary membrane, or ventilation-perfusion mismatch (ie, inadequate perfusion of ventilated parts of lung) or due to a right-to-left shunt. Hypoxemia due to all the previously mentioned causes except a shunt lesion is responsive to supplemental oxygen.

*References for this article can be found at*
https://doi.org/10.1542/pir.2020-002055

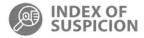

# INDEX OF SUSPICION

# Fatigue, Weight Loss, and Acute Chest Pain in a 15-year-old Boy

Madeline F.E. Parr, MD,* Katharine N. Clouser, MD, FAAP,* Meghan Tozzi, MD, FAAP,* Sejal M. Bhavsar, MD, FAAP*

*Joseph M. Sanzari Children's Hospital, Hackensack, NJ

## PRESENTATION

A 15-year-old boy with a history of membranous ventricular septal defect (VSD), not surgically repaired, presents to the emergency department (ED) with a 1-month history of fatigue, 5-lb (2.3-kg) weight loss, and productive cough, along with 3 days of right-sided chest pain. The patient went to his pediatrician approximately a month earlier due to cough, fatigue, and decreased activity and was presumed to have *Mycoplasma pneumoniae* and was treated empirically with azithromycin. His cough improved mildly, but he continued to have low energy. Two weeks before presentation, he developed night sweats without documented fever. Three days before presentation, the patient went to a gun range and was struck on his right chest by his rifle recoiling while he was shooting. After this event, he had constant chest pain and was taken to an orthopedic surgeon, where a chest radiograph was performed that, per verbal report, did not reveal evidence of fracture, and the patient's mother was not informed of any cardiopulmonary findings. His chest pain worsened with deep inspiration and he began having shortness of breath, which prompted his mother to bring him to the ED.

The patient denies any history of substance abuse or sexual activity, and he lives with his mother, father, and siblings. The family has had their home cleaned for the past 8 years by a housekeeper who had emigrated from El Salvador and developed an undiagnosed chronic cough 4 months ago. Travel history includes a trip to Florida 6 months ago, and he has traveled to Israel multiple times, with his most recent trip 3 years before presentation. He had COVID-19 pneumonia 3 months before presentation and did not require hospitalization. He received 2 doses of the Pfizer-BioNTech COVID-19 vaccine 3 weeks apart, with his second dose 2 months before presentation.

In the ED he appears fatigued but is afebrile and normotensive with normal heart and respiratory rates and is saturating at 98% on room air. He has mild right-sided chest wall tenderness overlying the T-4 level in the axillary line. He has decreased air entry to his bilateral lung bases, but no adventitious sounds are auscultated. He has a IV/VI harsh holosystolic murmur at Erb's point and is warm and well perfused, with peripheral pulses 2+ in all extremities. On oral examination he has braces on his upper and lower teeth and no evidence of caries or gingival inflammation. No lymphadenopathy, rash, abdominal tenderness, or organomegaly are appreciated. No evidence of cutaneous septic or vascular phenomena, such as Osler nodes, Janeway lesions, or nail bed hemorrhages, are appreciated.

AUTHOR DISCLOSURE: Drs Parr, Clouser, Tozzi, and Bhavsar have disclosed no financial relationships relevant to this article. This commentary does not contain a discussion of an unapproved/investigative use of a commercial product/device.

Laboratory results are significant for a white blood cell count of 9,900/μL (9.9 × 10⁹/L [reference range, 4,500–13,000/μL (4.5–13.0 × 10⁹/L)]) with a differential count of 73% neutrophils (reference range, 40%–62%), 15% lymphocytes (reference range, 27%–40%), 10% monocytes (reference range, 2%–8%); C-reactive protein level, 12.3 mg/dL (123 mg/L [reference range, <0.5 mg/dL (<5 mg/L)]); erythrocyte sedimentation rate, 99 mm/h (reference range, 0–15 mm/h); and hemoglobin level, 11.3 g/dL (113 g/L [reference range, 13.0–16.0 g/dL (130–160 g/L)]), with a mean corpuscular volume of 79.1 fL (reference range, 78–98 fL). A complete metabolic panel demonstrates normal serum levels of electrolytes and transaminases. His COVID-19 polymerase chain reaction, respiratory pathogen panel, rheumatoid factor, and antineutrophil cytoplasmic antibody panel are negative. His electrocardiogram demonstrates sinus arrhythmia with normal axis and intervals and normal voltages and repolarization. Two large-volume blood cultures at different peripheral sites are collected.

## DIFFERENTIAL DIAGNOSIS

The diagnostic possibilities included diverse infectious etiologies due to the patient's history and risk factors, including international and domestic travel, subacute fatigue, weight loss, night sweats, and acute chest pain. Differential diagnoses at the time of admission included pulmonary contusion, pneumothorax, pulmonary tuberculosis, multifocal pneumonia, sarcoidosis, endocarditis, distal infection with pulmonary septic emboli, and sequelae from COVID-19 infection. A chest radiograph demonstrated right middle lobe parenchymal infiltrate associated with right pleural effusion and possible left lower lobe pneumonia versus parenchymal contusion. A computed tomographic scan of the chest with contrast revealed multifocal consolidations most significant in the right middle lobe and left lower lobe. The consolidation in the left lower lobe demonstrated central necrosis, raising the suspicion for necrotizing pneumonia, pulmonary tuberculosis, lung abscesses, and septic emboli (Figs 1 and 2). Thoracic adenopathy was appreciated, and this constellation of findings suggested an infectious etiology rather than trauma.

The patient was started on ceftriaxone and placed on airborne isolation precautions due to concern for pulmonary tuberculosis. Early-morning sputum samples were collected for acid-fast bacilli smear and culture, and 3 consecutive morning samples had negative acid-fast bacilli smears. Interferon-γ release assay was negative, and the purified protein derivative was 0 mm. A transthoracic echocardiogram

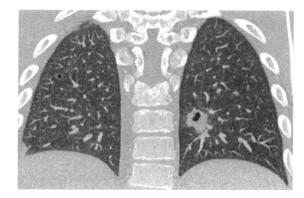

**Figure 1.** Apical computed tomographic view of the chest with consolidations in the left lower lung lobe and in the right middle lung lobe demonstrating central necrosis (red arrows).

(TTE) revealed a small, semimembranous VSD with minimal mitral regurgitation and no evidence of pedunculated vegetations. A transesophageal echocardiogram (TEE) was recommended to evaluate for small sessile lesions, but the family declined due to the more invasive nature of the study. After 72 hours of incubation, both initial blood cultures grew *Streptococcus mutans*, which is sensitive to ceftriaxone, penicillin G, and vancomycin. All blood cultures obtained after starting ceftriaxone treatment were negative. The patient was diagnosed as having *S mutans* endocarditis due to his positive blood cultures, historical cardiac defect, and evidence of septic emboli on chest imaging. He was treated with 6 weeks of ceftriaxone therapy. At his 4-week outpatient follow-up appointment, he continued to be afebrile and reported no complaints of chest pain, cough, or fatigue. Repeated chest radiography showed interval improvement of bilateral opacities.

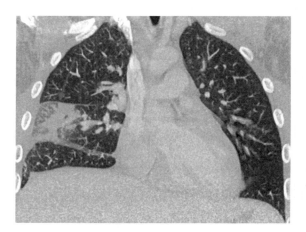

**Figure 2.** Apical computed tomographic view of the chest with a consolidation in the right middle lung lobe (red arrow). Motion artifact is present.

## DISCUSSION

Infective endocarditis (IE) is a rare diagnosis among pediatric patients in the United States, with an estimated incidence of 0.43 cases per 100,000 children compared with 15 cases per 100,000 adults. (1) Underlying cardiac malformations contribute significantly to the risk of IE, as approximately 53% of diagnosed cases are in children with congenital heart defects. (1) Disruptions in cardiac architecture from malformations such as atrial septal defects or VSDs create areas of increased flow in the heart chambers, which can damage the endocardium and increase the risk of platelet thrombus formation. (2) Platelet thrombi can subsequently be seeded in a state of transient bacteremia, leading to infectious thrombus formation. Due to bacteria hidden deep within a platelet thrombus, the treatment of IE typically requires 4 to 8 weeks of antibiotics to eradicate an infection. (2)

Diagnosis of IE is based on the modified Duke criteria, which has been adapted from the original Duke criteria. IE is categorized as definite, possible, or rejected based on pathologic, major, and minor clinical criteria. Definite diagnosis requires all subcriteria to be met within these categories, and possible diagnosis requires 2 major criteria, 1 major and 2 minor criteria, or 3 minor criteria. (3) The pathologic criteria are histologic confirmation of a cardiac or embolized vegetation or a cardiac lesion such as an abscess. Major criteria include evidence of endocardial involvement on imaging or a positive blood culture of an organism with a propensity for IE. Minor criteria are fever, predisposing cardiac lesion or drug use, immunologic phenomena, vascular phenomena such as septic emboli, or microbiological evidence of infection. Our patient's diagnosis of endocarditis was categorized as "possible" and relied on 3 minor criteria: his history of VSD, positive blood cultures, and the presence of multifocal pulmonary lesions that were attributed to septic emboli. Pulmonary septic emboli typically result from the showering of small bacterial thrombi from a central cardiac infectious thrombus. A TEE was recommended to confirm the diagnosis and to evaluate for sessile vegetations, but the family declined the more invasive test.

TEE demonstrates a significantly superior ability to diagnose endocarditis, with sensitivity of 94% compared with 24% with TTE among adults. (4) Many families can be hesitant to pursue TEE, but clinicians should consider strong recommendations of TEE in the setting of IE that may warrant additional intervention. Indications for considering surgical intervention include electrocardiographic conduction changes that would suggest abscess, significant change in valvular flow, children with prosthetic valves, or abnormalities of the thoracic cage or chest wall that make TTE less accurate. (2) Blood cultures are also highly important in the evaluation of IE, and 3 large-volume peripheral blood cultures drawn at different sites and under aseptic technique are preferred. Smaller volumes can be appropriate for smaller patients, such as 1 to 3 mL in infants or 5 to 7 mL in young children. (2)

IE can arise from a variety of infectious organisms. Staphylococcal IE continues to be the most frequently diagnosed subtype, but the incidence of streptococcal IE is increasing. (1) Among streptococcal infections, the viridans group of streptococci is most frequently identified. *S mutans* is a rare cause of endocarditis, primarily giving a subacute clinical picture, and can have significant morbidity and mortality. (5) *S mutans* is a bacterial species that is most frequently isolated in the oral cavity and can form biofilms that increase virulence. (6) Dental caries and poor oral hygiene contribute to the formation of *Streptococcus*-containing biofilms, which can predispose the host to transient bacteremia, as can routine dental brushing and flossing. (7) It is proposed that transient bacteremia, in conjunction with endocardial malformations seen in congenital heart defects, provides an environment for bacterial colonization, which can precipitate the development of subacute IE. (2) In a 4-year-old patient with *S mutans* IE, poor oral hygiene was determined to be the source of her bacteremia. (8) Although our patient had appropriate oral hygiene, he did have frequent orthodontic appointments for the management of braces, and it is possible that gingival manipulation during procedures or with daily oral care may have been the source of his bacteremia. In addition, before presentation, our patient was treated with a 5-day course of azithromycin, which likely partially treated the infection, accounting for his initial improvement of overall symptoms. Current guidelines do not recommend antibacterial prophylaxis against endocarditis for children with a VSD undergoing routine orthodontic care, as in our patient. (2) However, prophylaxis should be considered in high-risk children, such as those with cardiac transplants, previous cases of IE, cyanotic heart disease, or prosthetic valves.

### Lessons for the Clinician

- Infective endocarditis (IE) is a rare but vital differential diagnosis in pediatric patients presenting with subacute illness. Risk factors such as congenital heart malformation or poor oral hygiene should raise a clinician's suspicion for IE.
- The modified Duke criteria are favored in diagnosing IE in children. Transesophageal echocardiography should be performed when transthoracic echocardiography is

inadequate and when additional findings, such as an abscess, would change patient management.

- Staphylococcal species are most frequently implicated in IE, although streptococcal infections are on the rise.
- Peripheral blood cultures should be collected whenever IE is suspected, and 3 large-volume cultures at different sites and under aseptic technique should be collected at initial presentation. Blood cultures should be repeated within 24 to 48 hours of starting therapy.

*References for this article can be found at* https://doi.org/10.1542/pir.2022-005552.

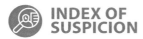

# Fever and Pleuritic Chest Pain in a 16-year-old Girl with Ulcerative Colitis

Michael Chmielewski, MD,* Jessica VanNostrand, MD,† Matthew Hollander, MD, MHA†

*University of Vermont Larner College of Medicine, Burlington, VT
†Vermont Children's Hospital, Burlington, VT

## PRESENTATION

A 16-year-old girl with a history of asthma, ulcerative colitis (UC), allergic rhinitis, multiple food and environmental allergies, migraines, and autoimmune hypothyroidism presents to the emergency department with 2 days of worsening chest pain. She describes the pain as a sharp sensation localized to her left upper chest, which is exacerbated by deep inhalation. Review of systems is notable for 3 days of intermittent low-grade fevers and a dry cough, which has not improved with inhaled albuterol or fluticasone use. On physical examination the patient is pale. Her respiratory rate is elevated to 22 breaths/min, with oxygen saturation greater than 95% on room air. Her temperature is 101°F (38.3°C), heart rate is 130 beats/min, and blood pressure is 122/79 mm Hg. Her height is 64 in (162.8 cm) (51st percentile), weight is 114.6 lb (52 kg) (40th percentile), and BMI is 19.6. A thorough physical examination is performed, which is notable for marked nasal edema and copious clear discharge bilaterally. A systolic grade III/VI cardiac murmur is auscultated, and breath sounds are clear bilaterally without evidence of respiratory distress. On abdominal examination bowel sounds are hyperactive. There is diffuse abdominal tenderness to palpation without rebound tenderness or palpable masses. No rashes are identified.

She was diagnosed as having UC 8 months before the current presentation after 7 months of abdominal pain and diarrhea. Colonoscopy at the time of UC diagnosis was notable for pancolitis with widespread edema and mucosal friability. Surgical pathologic testing of her colon biopsy sample obtained during colonoscopy revealed widespread cryptitis, crypt abscesses, crypt destruction and repair, and widespread superficial mucosal injury and repair, consistent with UC. There were no granulomas noted on the pathology sample, and a terminal ilium biopsy specimen was notable for scattered intraepithelial eosinophils focally. In the 8 months after the patient's diagnosis of UC, her gastrointestinal (GI) symptoms were poorly controlled with mesalamine and oral corticosteroids. Infliximab was initiated 1 month before this presentation due to worsening abdominal pain, bloody diarrhea, and a 15-lb (6.8-kg, or 10%) weight loss over 6 months.

Scheduled medications at the time of presentation include infliximab infusions, mesalamine, levothyroxine, cholecalciferol, coenzyme Q10, cyanocobalamin, magnesium, lactobacillus cultures, inhaled fluticasone-salmeterol, and a 2-week course of ciprofloxacin and metronidazole for diarrhea. The patient recently discontinued taking oral budesonide and montelukast. Medications taken

**AUTHOR DISCLOSURE:** Drs Chmielewski, VanNostrand, and Hollander have disclosed no financial relationships relevant to this article. This commentary does not contain a discussion of an unapproved/investigative use of a commercial product/device.

Dr Chmielewski's current affiliation is University of Minnesota, Minneapolis, MN.

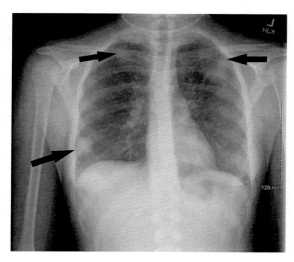

**Figure 1.** Chest radiograph demonstrating multifocal nodular airspace opacities seen in the right lower lobe, left upper lung, and right lung apex (arrows).

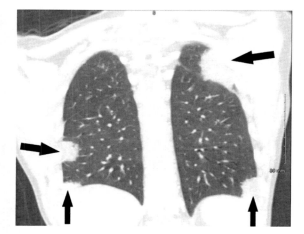

**Figure 2.** Coronal computed tomographic scan of the thoracic cavity demonstrating multiple regions of peripheral airspace opacity (arrows).

as needed include ibuprofen, inhaled albuterol, cetirizine, ondansetron, sumatriptan, intranasal fluticasone, and intranasal azelastine.

A chest radiograph reveals multifocal nodular airspace opacities in the right upper, right lower, and left lower lobes with an otherwise normal cardiothymic silhouette (Fig 1). Nasal endoscopy reveals boggy nasal mucosa without granulomas. The electrocardiogram and echocardiogram are normal. Laboratory results are notable for an elevated white blood cell count of 15,000/μL (15.0 × 10⁹/L) (reference range, 4,600–11,200/μL [4.6–11.2 × 10⁹/L]) with a newly elevated eosinophil count of 2,460/μL (2.46 × 10⁹/L) (reference range, 30–610/μL [0.03–0.61 × 10⁹/L]), or 16.2% (reference range, 0%-6%) on the differential count. Erythrocyte sedimentation rate is elevated at 28 mm/hour (reference range, <20 mm/hour), and C-reactive protein level is elevated at 2.3 mg/dL (23.3 mg/L) (reference range, <1.0 mg/dL [<10.0 mg/L]). Hemoglobin level is 10.9 g/dL (109 g/L) (reference range, 12.0–16.0 g/dL [120–160 g/L]), hematocrit level is 34.1% (reference range, 36%–46%), and platelet count is 711 × 10³/μL (711 × 10⁹/L) (reference range, 156–312 × 10³/μL [156–312 × 10⁹/L]). Antinuclear antibody is positive at 1:160 (reference range, <1:40–1:160), and perinuclear antinuclear cytoplasmic antibody (p-ANCA) is positive at 1:2,560 (reference range, <1:40). Immunoglobulin E (IgE) level is elevated at 60.5 mg/dL (6.05 × 10⁴ mg/L) (reference range, <3.79 × 10⁴ mg/L). A bronchoalveolar lavage is notable for 75% neutrophils with negative testing for fungi, acid-fast bacilli, bacteria, aspergillus, and cytomegalovirus. Magnetic resonance enterography of the abdomen reveals pancolitis with thickened large bowel walls and increased contrast

enhancement. Chest computed tomography (CT) (Fig 2) confirms multiple regions of peripheral airspace opacity, as well as diffuse bronchovascular thickening and enlarged hilar lymph nodes. Histopathologic analysis of a CT-guided lung nodule biopsy demonstrates extravascular eosinophilic inflammation and foamy macrophages suggestive of nonnecrotizing granulomas.

## DISCUSSION

### Differential Diagnosis

This 16-year-old female patient presents with pleuritic chest pain, fever, and multifocal airspace opacities in the setting of poorly controlled UC and peripheral eosinophilia. The differential diagnosis includes infections such as viral or bacterial pneumonia, pulmonary tuberculosis, allergic pulmonary aspergillosis, malignancy, and vasculitis. Preceding immunosuppression in the form of oral corticosteroids and infliximab infusions increases the risk of opportunistic infections. Pulmonary infiltrates raise suspicion for neoplastic processes, including lymphoma and eosinophilic leukemia. Hypereosinophilia, defined as a serum eosinophil count greater than 1,500/μL (1.5 × 10⁹/L), is a prominent feature in this case. Hypereosinophilic syndromes, defined by the association of hypereosinophilia with eosinophil-mediated organ damage or dysfunction, are considered in the differential diagnosis. The patient was previously treated with mesalamine for her UC, a medication associated with eosinophilic pneumonia (EP). (1) Likewise, EP can accompany other connective tissue diseases, including eosinophilic fasciitis, systemic lupus erythematosus, and several rare immunodeficiencies, including hyper-IgE syndrome. Infliximab is an anti–tumor necrosis factor α monoclonal antibody that has also been associated with development of vasculitis. (2) Granulomatosis with polyangiitis (GPA), an ANCA-positive vasculitis, can present with upper or lower airway granulomas.

## Actual Diagnosis

The patient fulfills the American College of Rheumatology classification criteria (3) for diagnosing eosinophilic GPA (EGPA). EGPA is diagnosed with the presence of 4 or more of the following 6 criteria: 1) history of asthma; 2) eosinophilia greater than 10% on the white blood cell differential count; 3) mononeuropathy or polyneuropathy; 4) nonfixed pulmonary infiltrates; 5) paranasal sinus abnormality (history of acute or chronic paranasal sinus pain, tenderness, or radiographic opacification of the paranasal sinuses); and 6) extravascular eosinophils observed on biopsy specimen. (3) This patient met 5 of the 6 criteria with her history of asthma, peripheral eosinophilia to 16%, history of chronic allergic rhinitis, nonfixed pulmonary infiltrates observed on CT scan, and extravascular eosinophils observed on pulmonary biopsy.

## The Condition

EGPA (formerly known as Churg-Strauss syndrome) is a small- and medium-sized vessel vasculitis characterized by eosinophil-rich necrotizing granulomas that typically affect the respiratory tract. (4) EGPA constitutes a rare form of vasculitis in adults and children, with approximately 106 pediatric cases reported in the literature to date, mainly in individual case reports. (5) EPGA is a multisystem inflammatory disorder that commonly presents with asthma, pulmonary eosinophilic infiltrates, nasal polyposis, and allergic rhinosinusitis. (4) Other manifestations include peripheral neuropathy (usually in the form of mononeuritis multiplex), subcutaneous nodules and purpura secondary to leukocytoclastic vasculitis, gastroenteritis, glomerulonephritis, and cardiac involvement. (4) Laboratory findings typically include marked hypereosinophilia, increased inflammatory markers, and ANCA positivity (typically p-ANCA), with histopathologic analysis notable for extravascular necrotizing eosinophilic granulomas and small/medium vessel vasculitis with fibrinoid necrosis. (4) No pediatric-specific diagnostic criteria have been validated. Nomenclature published in 2013 describes case definitions, not classification or diagnostic criteria, commonly used in pediatric clinical trials. (6) EGPA is distinguished from other ANCA-positive vasculitides, including GPA, in that the latter is more often positive for c-ANCA, does not demonstrate peripheral eosinophilia or eosinophilic inflammation on histologic tissue examination, and often presents with distinctive upper airway involvement, including nasal granulomas, erosions, or crusting. (7)

Although rare, vasculitis may co-occur with inflammatory bowel disease (IBD), with a specific association between EGPA and UC. (8)(9) EGPA has been reported to occur with UC more often than with Crohn disease, with EGPA and UC both often positive for p-ANCA. (4)(8)(9)(10) In contrast, Crohn disease is often p-ANCA negative. (10) Furthermore, EGPA and UC are both Th2-mediated diseases, with a possible shared pathophysiology between the two involving interleukin-5 (IL-5). (9) In EGPA, increased levels of IL-5 have been demonstrated in flares, with secretion by Th2 lymphocytes recruiting eosinophils to peripheral tissues. (9) In UC, Th2 lymphocytes in the lamina propria secrete IL-5, which may also increase the number of eosinophils in the intestinal mucosa during active UC. (9) In patients with coexisting IBD and ANCA-associated vasculitis, IBD typically predates the onset of vasculitis. (8) However, because EGPA can manifest with GI symptoms, it may be difficult to distinguish between IBD and EGPA. Small vessel vasculitis may mimic IBD during the eosinophilic stage of the disease, which is characterized by granulomatous inflammation of the GI mucosa. (7)(8)

This patient was diagnosed as having EGPA after being treated for biopsy-confirmed UC for 8 months. This case was challenging in that EGPA developed after the diagnosis of UC with GI symptoms similar to the patient's previous UC flares. In a systematic review and longitudinal study evaluating the association between IBD and small vessel vasculitis, Sy et al (8) excluded patients who had been diagnosed as having vasculitis less than 12 months after the onset of IBD due to potential misdiagnosis of GI manifestations of vasculitis as IBD. However, exclusive presentation with vasculitis involving the GI tract is rare, and GI vasculitis typically presents with gastroduodenal or colorectal ulcerations on endoscopy. (7) In addition, Hokama et al (11) observed patchy mucosal erythema and mild infiltration of eosinophils around crypts in a patient with EGPA and GI involvement. In contrast, our patient had contiguous pancolitis at the time of UC diagnosis with colonic crypt abscesses devoid of eosinophils on histologic examination. Thus, we propose that this patient developed EGPA 8 months after being diagnosed as having UC through a shared inflammatory mechanism between these distinct disease entities.

A complexity of this case was the fact that her pulmonary biopsy revealed nonnecrotizing granulomas, in contrast to usual classification criteria. This detail was reviewed at length with pathology department staff, who agreed that the presence of granulomas was supportive of EGPA despite the absence of necrotic tissue. In addition, our patient's autoimmune thyroid disease was well controlled for many years at the time of this diagnosis, so we do not feel that it was a confounding factor in the course above. Autoimmune thyroid disease is associated with other autoimmune organ-specific diseases, such as type 1 diabetes; Addison, celiac, and systemic diseases, including ANCA vasculitis (12)(13)(14); systemic lupus erythematosus; and Sjögren syndrome.

Given this patient's peripheral and pulmonary interstitial eosinophilia, we considered mesalamine as a potential cause of drug-induced EP. In a review of case reports of drug-induced acute and chronic EP, mesalamine was one of the most common drugs implicated. (1) However, our patient had stopped taking mesalamine almost 2 months before presentation, and the pattern of bronchovascular thickening and nonfixed nodules is characteristic for neither acute nor chronic EP. It is also unlikely that the patient developed EGPA 1 month after initiation of infliximab therapy for poorly controlled UC. In a retrospective review, Sokumbi et al (2) described 8 patients who developed vasculitis after treatment with anti–tumor necrosis factor α agents for a mean of 34 months, considerably longer than the patient herein. These patients presented with cutaneous small vessel vasculitis (63%), neuropathy (25%), and renal involvement (13%), and no pulmonary involvement was observed. (2) Histopathologic specimens obtained were diagnostic for leukocytoclastic vasculitis in those with cutaneous involvement, perivascular and perineural inflammation in those with neuropathy, and mild IgA nephropathy in patients with renal involvement. (2)

## Management

Management of EGPA typically consists of an induction phase with tapered corticosteroids and corticosteroid-sparing agents, such as cyclophosphamide, for quickly controlling disease activity. Induction is followed by maintenance therapy with immunosuppression to achieve remission. (4) There is much overlap in corticosteroid-sparing immunomodulation choices for IBD and EGPA, including methotrexate, azathioprine, infliximab, and rituximab. The evolving evidence base for EGPA explores monoclonal antibodies against various targets, such as IgE (omalizumab) (15) and IL-5 (mepolizumab). (16)

## Patient Course

The patient was treated with an initial prednisone taper and cyclophosphamide infusions for 3 months for induction. She was successfully transitioned to azathioprine for maintenance therapy. Her cough and pleuritic chest pain resolved with normalization of inflammatory markers, and she has regained weight. She has achieved disease remission from both EGPA and UC for longer than 1 year to date.

## Lessons for the Clinician

- Eosinophilic granulomatosis with polyangiitis constitutes a rare form of pediatric vasculitis.
- Inflammatory bowel disease and vasculitis may rarely co-occur, likely through a shared inflammatory pathway. (5)
- In patients with multisystem complaints, it is important to consider both gastrointestinal manifestations of inflammatory bowel disease and systemic vasculitis in the differential diagnosis.

*References for this article can be found at*
https://doi.org/10.1542/pir.2021-004937.

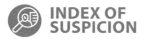

INDEX OF
SUSPICION

# Fever and Shock in a 17-month-old Girl

Niharika Samtani, MD,* Jennifer S. Kicker, MD,* Jennifer C. Geracht, MD,* Matthew D. Eberly, MD†

*Division of Pediatric Critical Care, Department of Pediatrics, and
†Department of Pediatrics, Walter Reed National Military Medical Center, Bethesda, MD

## PRESENTATION

A 17-month-old term, previously healthy, fully vaccinated girl presents to the emergency department (ED) with a 5-day history of poor oral intake, fever, and lethargy. Four days earlier she presented to an urgent care facility, where results of influenza and severe acute respiratory syndrome coronavirus 2 (SARS-CoV-2) polymerase chain reaction (PCR) testing were negative. She was discharged with instructions for supportive care. Her symptoms persisted, prompting a second visit where again she was discharged with similar instructions. Symptoms failed to resolve; therefore, her parents brought her to the ED for further evaluation.

Review of systems is negative for rhinorrhea, cough, vomiting, diarrhea, foul-smelling urine, rash, peeling skin, conjunctival injection, and lymphadenopathy. She lives at home with her parents, older siblings, and grandparents. They reside in the Mid-Atlantic United States and deny recent travel. She has not had much outdoor exposure or any known contact with animals. The patient attends indoor church services with her family; she is unable to accommodate a face mask due to age. There are no child care exposures or recent sick contacts; however, multiple members of the household experienced chills and fatigue 4 weeks before presentation. Her father underwent SARS-CoV-2 PCR testing at that time and was negative.

ED presentation vital signs are as follows: temperature, 101.3°F (38.5°C); respiratory rate, 50 breaths/min; heart rate, 170 beats/min; blood pressure, 72/38 mm Hg; and oxygen saturation, 90% in room air. Her examination is significant for labored breathing, tachycardia, poor peripheral perfusion, cold extremities, and lethargy. There is no rash. Cardiac examination reveals regular rhythm without murmurs, gallop, or rub. Her abdomen is nondistended without hepatosplenomegaly.

She is volume resuscitated and provided vasoactive support via intraosseous access. Initial urinalysis is concentrated and reveals pyuria. Blood and urine cultures are sent, and antibiotics are initiated. She is intubated due to concern for progressive shock as evidenced by continued poor perfusion, oliguria, and lethargy. She is transferred to the PICU on ventilator support.

On arrival, venous and arterial access is obtained and blood work is collected (Table). Due to an increase of SARS-CoV-2 caseload in the community at the time, a history of flulike illness circulating in the home, and features of shock on presentation, further laboratory studies are obtained, including pro–brain-type natriuretic peptide, high-sensitivity troponin T, C-reactive protein (CRP), interleukin-6 (IL-6), procalcitonin, erythrocyte sedimentation rate, ferritin, fibrinogen, coagulation profile, respiratory pathogen PCR swab, and serum viral studies, including an immunoglobulin profile for antibodies to SARS-CoV-2. Urine microscopy shows greater

**AUTHOR DISCLOSURE:** Drs Samtani, Kicker, Geracht, and Eberly have disclosed no financial relationships relevant to this article. This commentary does not contain a discussion of an unapproved/investigative use of a commercial product/device.

*The views expressed in this article are those of the authors and do not reflect the official policy of the Department of Army/Navy/Air Force, Department of Defense, or US Government.*

**Table.** Laboratory Evaluation

| LABORATORY FINDING | REFERENCE RANGE | VALUE AT PICU PRESENTATION |
|---|---|---|
| pH (arterial) | 7.35–7.45 | 7.313[a] |
| Pao$_2$ (arterial), mm Hg (kPa) (PEEP, 5 cmH$_2$O; Fio$_2$, 40%) | 83–108 (11.04–14.36) | 153 (20.35)[a] |
| Pco$_2$ (arterial), mm Hg (kPa) (SIMV, pressure control [peak inspiratory pressure 24] with volume guarantee, plus pressure support [10cm H$_2$0/5cm H$_2$0]; rate, 35) | 27–40 (3.59–5.32) | 33.4 (4.44) |
| Bicarbonate (arterial), mEq/L (mmol/L) | 22–26 (22–26) | 16.9 (16.9)[a] |
| Base excess (arterial), mEq/L (mmol/L) | –2 to 2 (–2 to 2) | –9 (–9)[a] |
| Lactate (arterial), mg/dL (mmol/L) | 4.5–9.01 (0.5–1.0) | 14.41 (1.6)[a] |
| Sodium, mEq/L (mmol/L) | 136–145 (136–145) | 135 (135)[a] |
| Potassium, mEq/L (mmol/L) | 3.5–5.1 (3.5–5.1) | 4.0 (4.0) |
| Chloride, mEq/L (mmol/L) | 98–107 (98–107) | 104 (104) |
| Carbon dioxide, mEq/L (mmol/L) | 22–29 (22–29) | 15 (15)[a] |
| Blood urea nitrogen, mg/dL (mmol/L) | 4–19 (1.43–6.78) | 41.9 (14.96)[a] |
| Creatinine, mg/dL (µmol/L) | 0.3–0.7 (26.52–61.88) | 1.05 (92.82)[a] |
| Glucose, mg/dL (mmol/L) | 74–106 (4.11–5.88) | 282 (15.65)[a] |
| Albumin, g/dL (g/L) | 3.5–5.2 (35–52) | 2.4 (24)[a] |
| Aspartate aminotransferase, U/L (µkat/L) | 13–35 (0.22–0.58) | 35 (0.58) |
| Alanine aminotransferase, U/L (µkat/L) | 5–45 (0.08–0.75) | 88 (1.47)[a] |
| White blood cells, /µL (×10$^9$/L) | 6,000–17,000 (6–17) | 39,000 (39)[a] |
| Neutrophils, % | 17–74 | 73.9 |
| Bands, % | 0–10 | 16.6[a] |
| Lymphocytes, % | 27–80 | 7.5[a] |
| Hemoglobin, g/dL (g/L) | 10.5–13.5 (105–135) | 8.1 (81)[a] |
| Hematocrit, % | 33–39 | 26[a] |
| Mean corpuscular volume, µm$^3$ (fL) | 70–86 (70–86) | 87 (87)[a] |
| Platelets, ×10$^3$/µL (×10$^9$/L) | 150–550 (150–550) | 169 (169) |
| Pro–brain-type natriuretic peptide, pg/mL (ng/L) | 5–125 (5–125) | >70,000 (>70,000)[a] |
| High-sensitivity troponin T, ng/mL (µg/L) | 0–0.019 (0–0.019) | 0.0592 (0.0592)[a] |
| C-reactive protein, mg/dL (mg/L) | 0–0.6 (0–6) | 26.2 (262)[a] |
| Procalcitonin, ng/mL (ng/L) | 0–0.25 (0–250) | 23.53 (23,530)[a] |
| Ferritin, ng/mL (µg/L) | 7–140 (7–140) | 515 (515)[a] |
| Erythrocyte sedimentation rate, mm/hr | 2–34 | 29 |
| Interleukin-6, pg/mL | 0–13 | 352[ab] |
| D-dimer, µg/mL (nmol/L) | 0–0.49(0–2.68) | 10.7 (1.95)[a] |
| Fibrinogen, mg/dL (g/L) | 207–454 (6.09–13.35) | 519 (15.26)[a] |
| Prothrombin time, s | 11.8–14.6 | 16.5[a] |
| International normalized ratio | 2.0–4.5 | 1.3[a] |
| Partial thromboplastin time, s | 23.8–35.5 | 41.7[a] |
| SARS-CoV-2 IgM | Negative | Negative[c] |
| SARS-CoV-2 IgG | Negative | Positive[ac] |
| Respiratory pathogen swab | | |
|   Influenza A, B, and C | Negative | Negative |
|   Respiratory syncytial virus | Negative | Negative |
|   *Mycoplasma pneumoniae* | Negative | Negative |
|   *Bordetella parapertussis* | Negative | Negative |
|   *Bordetella pertussis* | Negative | Negative |
|   Adenovirus | Negative | Negative |
|   Coronaviruses 229E/HKU1/NL63/OC43 | Negative | Negative |
|   Metapneumovirus | Negative | Negative |
|   Parainfluenza 1/2/3/4 | Negative | Negative |
|   Rhinovirus/enterovirus | Negative | Negative |
|   SARS-COV-2 | Negative | Negative |

Fio$_2$=fraction of inspired oxygen, Ig=immunoglobulin, PEEP=positive end-expiratory pressure, SARS-CoV-2=severe acute respiratory syndrome coronavirus 2, SIMV=synchronized intermittent mandatory ventilation.
[a]Value is outside the reference range.
[b]Send out laboratory drawn on admission, results received on hospital day 5.
[c]Send out laboratory drawn on admission, results received on hospital day 6.

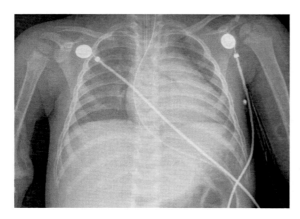

**Figure.** Chest radiograph demonstrating patchy perihilar opacities without cardiomegaly.

than 40 red blood cells per high-power field [reference range 0-2], 11 to 20 white blood cells per high-power field [reference range 0-2], and moderate bacteria [none] concerning for urosepsis. Complete metabolic profile reveals acute kidney injury and mild liver inflammation. Complete blood cell count shows leukocytosis and a depressed lymphocyte count. She has a mild anemia with a normal platelet count. Levels of pro–brain-type natriuretic peptide and high-sensitivity troponin T are elevated. CRP, procalcitonin, ferritin, fibrinogen, and D-dimer levels are high. Coagulation studies are largely within normal limits. Respiratory pathogen panel is negative. A lumbar puncture is performed, and the cerebrospinal fluid is significant for a white blood cell count of 74/μL (0.074 × 10$^9$/L) [reference range 6-17], a glucose level of 176 mg/dL (9.77 mmol/L) (reference range, 60–80 mg/dL [3.33–4.44 mmol/L]), and a negative Gram-stain.

Her chest radiograph (Fig) demonstrates patchy perihilar opacities without cardiomegaly. Echocardiography is performed and shows a dilated left ventricle, moderately decreased systolic function (ejection fraction of 45%) with moderate-severe mitral regurgitation, and diastolic dysfunction; coronary arteries are within normal limits.

## DISCUSSION

### Differential Diagnosis

A differential diagnosis for hemodynamic compromise/shock in a child with fever and elevated inflammatory markers includes sepsis, toxic shock syndrome, myocarditis, or a postinfectious hyperinflammatory condition, including the multisystem inflammatory syndrome in children (MIS-C) related to SARS-CoV-2.

Shock is an altered pathophysiologic state in which an imbalance of oxygen supply versus demand leads to tissue hypoxia. If not appropriately recognized and supported,

the shock syndrome can rapidly advance to end organ damage and death. Four broad categories of shock in pediatrics include hypovolemic, cardiogenic, distributive, and obstructive, with the entity of septic shock demonstrating overlapping features. Hypovolemic shock results from a decrease in preload due to fluid loss with reduced stroke volume, decreased cardiac output (CO), and a compensatory increase in systemic vascular resistance (SVR). Cardiogenic shock results from an impairment of the cardiac pump with reduction in CO, clinical signs and symptoms of volume overload, as well as a compensatory increase in SVR. Distributive or vasodilatory shock results from an abnormal distribution of blood flow with a decrease in SVR leading to a functional hypovolemia. Obstructive shock is the sequalae of a physical obstruction to blood flow/CO with a compensatory increase in SVR. This patient demonstrated the overlapping features of hypovolemic and cardiogenic shock likely in the setting of septic shock. Although initial management and stabilization progresses down a common pathway with intravascular volume resuscitation, vasoactive support, and reduction of metabolic demand, understanding and identification of shock type with formulation of a differential diagnosis and recognition of etiology will help guide targeted management. For example, treatment for sepsis may prompt consideration of toxic shock syndrome and rickettsial diseases with initiation of broad-spectrum antibiotics, including ceftriaxone, vancomycin, +/− clindamycin, and doxycycline. Treatment for cardiogenic shock from myocarditis or MIS-C would warrant administration of intravenous immunoglobulins, with the latter possibly benefiting from the addition of glucocorticoids and other adjunctive immunomodulating agents.

### The Condition

Although case definition criteria for MIS-C vary between health agencies, the Centers for Disease Control and Prevention (CDC) defines this as a clinically severe illness requiring hospitalization in an individual younger than 21 years presenting with fever for 24 hours or more, with laboratory evidence of inflammation and multisystem organ involvement, no plausible alternative diagnosis, and evidence of current or recent SARS-CoV-2 infection (PCR, serology, or antigen test) or exposure to a suspected or confirmed COVID-19 case within 4 weeks before onset of symptoms. Laboratory evidence of inflammation includes 1 or more of the following: elevated CRP level, erythrocyte sedimentation rate, fibrinogen level, procalcitonin level, D-dimer level, ferritin level, lactate dehydrogenase level, IL-6 level, or neutrophil count or reduced lymphocyte count or albumin level. Most children with MIS-C have an antibody response favoring immunoglobulin (Ig) G over IgM with a low or absent nasopharyngeal viral load suggesting a postinfectious phenomenon. (1)

Although the MIS-C phenotype may overlap with Kawasaki disease and macrophage activation syndrome, it seems to have a distinct pathophysiology based on unique inflammatory/immunologic features such as markedly elevated IL-6 level, moderately elevated ferritin level, and evidence of lymphopenia. (2) In contrast to the typical Kawasaki disease cohort, the MIS-C population tends to be older, with a median age at presentation of 9 to 10 years. (2)(3) Black and Hispanic children seem to be disproportionately affected. (4)(5)(6) Clinically, patients with MIS-C present with cardiac manifestations distinct from Kawasaki disease, namely, abnormal ventricular function frequently requiring vasoactive support. (2)(7)(8) Typical noncardiovascular involvement has been described to include predominantly gastrointestinal and mucocutaneous manifestations. (5) Without a high index of suspicion and targeted evaluation, MIS-C can be overlooked in a younger population presenting with isolated fever and shock.

## Diagnosis

In the case of this 17-month-old presenting in shock, with a preceding 5-day history of fever and lethargy in the absence of gastrointestinal and dermatologic features on presentation, one needed a high level of suspicion for the diagnosis of MIS-C. At the time of PICU admission she demonstrated generalized inflammation, hemodynamic compromise, and multisystem organ involvement. There was initial suspicion for urosepsis with pyuria and bacteriuria on urinalysis; however, final urine, blood, and cerebrospinal fluid cultures remained negative. Later in her hospital course, SARS-CoV-2 IgG was noted to be positive and IgM negative; IL-6 level was found to be markedly elevated. With these data, we are led to a presumptive diagnosis of MIS-C.

## Patient Course/Management

The patient received ongoing fluid resuscitation and vasoactive support. She remained intubated and sedated to minimize metabolic demand and to maintain invasive line and endotracheal tube safety. Cultures were obtained and she was started on ceftriaxone and vancomycin to provide coverage against *Staphylococcus aureus*, group A streptococcus, and pneumococcus. Clindamycin was added for antitoxin effect. Pediatric cardiology, infectious disease, and rheumatology were consulted on hospital day 1. Echocardiography revealed reduced left ventricle function

without coronary artery involvement. Viral serologies were sent before treatment with intravenous immunoglobulins for concern of myocarditis. Stress dose hydrocortisone was started in the setting of fluid- and catecholamine-resistant shock. Milrinone was added for afterload reduction in the setting of continued cardiac dysfunction. Vasoactive support was weaned as her hemodynamics stabilized and lactate levels cleared. Furosemide and spironolactone were administered for diuresis with intermittent electrolyte repletion. Antibiotics were discontinued after 48 hours when cultures showed no bacterial growth. Anakinra, an IL-1 antagonist, was initiated per pediatric rheumatology recommendations in the setting of rising inflammatory markers and concern for an evolving cytokine storm phenomenon. (9) She was liberated from the ventilator by hospital day 3. Echocardiography continued to show improved function sparing the coronaries; she was transitioned from milrinone to an angiotensin-converting enzyme inhibitor and low-dose aspirin for prophylactic coronary protection. As inflammatory markers showed a downward trend, she transitioned from intravenous hydrocortisone to oral prednisolone. On hospital day 6, SARS-CoV-2 serologies were reported; IgM was negative and IgG was positive, indicating past infection. By hospital day 7 she was transferred to the general floor and was subsequently discharged on hospital day 11. She was maintained on anakinra, enalapril, aspirin, and prednisolone with pediatric rheumatology and cardiology follow-up for immunomodulatory therapy titration and serial cardiac assessment.

## LESSONS FOR THE CLINICIAN

- It is important to entertain a broad differential diagnosis when caring for a pediatric patient in shock. Although initial management and stabilization will overlap, consideration of etiology will help guide subsequent management.
- Although most patients with multisystem inflammatory syndrome in children tend to be school-age with gastrointestinal and/or mucocutaneous symptoms, it is important to have a high index of suspicion and consider this etiology even in younger children presenting with isolated fever and hemodynamic compromise.
- In cases of undifferentiated shock, it is important to engage multidisciplinary expertise early, including pediatric intensive care, cardiology, infectious disease, and rheumatology.

*References for this article can be found at*
https://doi.org/10.1542/pir.2021-005090.

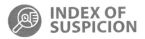

INDEX OF
SUSPICION

# Neonate with Respiratory Distress, Bilateral Microtia, Hypocalcemia, and Lymphopenia

Leela R. Patel, MD,* Brittany C. Flemming, MD,* Katrina A. Savioli, MD, FAAP*

*Department of Pediatrics, Walter Reed National Military Medical Center, Bethesda, MD

## PRESENTATION

A 2-day-old term boy is transferred to a tertiary NICU for further diagnostic evaluation and management of respiratory failure. His prenatal course was normal. Delivery was complicated by prolonged rupture of membranes with arrest of labor, necessitating cesarean delivery. During resuscitation, respiratory distress with stridor, retractions, and poor color were noted, followed by bradycardia. A 6-French nasal suction catheter could not be advanced through either nare; however, an orogastric tube was passed into the stomach without difficulty. Positive pressure ventilation was performed and demonstrated success only after the mouth was opened. Due to continued hypoxemia and stridor, a laryngeal mask airway was placed. Apgar scores were 3 and 7 at 1 and 5 minutes of life, respectively. The infant was admitted to the special care nursery of a community hospital for stabilization before transfer to the NICU.

On NICU admission, oral endotracheal intubation is successfully performed. Vital signs on admission are as follows: temperature, 99.5°F (37.5°C); heart rate, 147 beats/min; respiratory rate, 51 breaths/min; blood pressure, 76/54 mm Hg; and oxygen saturation, 100% on minimal conventional mechanical ventilator settings (synchronized intermittent mandatory ventilation/pressure support mode with tidal volume of 5 mL/kg; maximum inspiratory pressure, 25 cm $H_2O$; positive end-expiratory pressure, 5 cm $H_2O$; respiratory rate, 30 breaths/min; and fraction of inspired oxygen, 21%). Physical examination on admission is notable for ear asymmetry with bilateral dysmorphic microtia (Fig 1), intermittent stridor before intubation with clear lung sounds bilaterally after intubation, and borderline microphallus (stretched penile length of 2.2 cm). Eye examination reveals equal pupils responsive to light without abnormalities of the irises; fundoscopy is not performed on admission. Cardiac examination findings are within normal limits, without murmur, and with normal femoral pulses. Abdominal examination discloses a soft, nontender, nondistended abdomen without organomegaly. Neurologic examination is limited in the setting of intubation but reveals an alert infant with normal tone for gestational age, equal movements of all extremities, and intact palmar grasp bilaterally. Skin examination findings are normal, without rashes or lesions.

Laboratory values (reference ranges) are notable for significant hypocalcemia, with an ionized calcium level of 3 mg/dL (0.75 mmol/L) (3.9–6.0 mg/dL [0.97–1.50 mmol/L]) and a serum calcium level of 5.5 mg/dL (1.3 mmol/L) (9–11 mg/dL [2.25–2.75 mmol/L]); hyperphosphatemia, with a phosphorus level of

AUTHOR DISCLOSURE Drs Patel, Flemming, and Savioli have no financial disclosures relevant to this article. This commentary does not contain a discussion of an unapproved/investigative use of a commercial product/device.

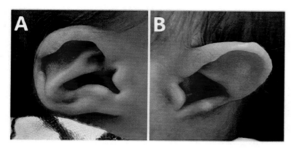

**Figure 1.** Dysmorphic ears of the patient, which are characteristic of CHARGE (coloboma, heart defects, atresia choanae, growth retardation, genital abnormalities, and ear abnormalities) syndrome. A. Square-shaped right ear with prominent antihelix and hypoplastic lobule. B. Left ear with decreased cartilage, an aplastic lobule, and a triangular concha.

8.5 mg/dL (2.75 mmol/L) (4.0–6.5 mg/dL [1.29–2.10 mmol/L]); a normal white blood cell count of 17,500/μL (17.5 × 10$^9$/L) (9,400–34,000/μL [9.4–34.0 × 10$^9$/L]); and lymphopenia, with an absolute lymphocyte count of 1,575/μL (1.575 × 10$^9$/L) (5,000/μL [5.0 × 10$^9$/L]; 95% confidence interval, 2,000–17,000/μL [2–17 × 10$^9$/L]). Further evaluation reveals a low intact parathyroid hormone level of 8.9 pg/mL (8.9 ng/L) (reference range, 15–65 pg/mL [15–65 ng/L]) with a normal serum 25-hydroxyvitamin D level of 26.6 ng/mL (66.39 nmol/L) (reference range, >20 ng/mL [>49.92 nmol/L]). Newborn metabolic screening is expedited and reveals undetectable T-cell receptor excision circles (TRECs).

Chest radiography shows a small, hypoplastic thymus and 11 paired ribs and is otherwise normal, with a normal cardiac silhouette. Initial echocardiography shows suprasystemic right ventricular pressures with mild right ventricular hypertrophy and mild pulmonary artery branch stenosis but no structural lesions. The aortic arch is leftward with a normal branching pattern.

## DISCUSSION

### Differential Diagnosis

CHARGE (coloboma, heart defects, atresia choanae, growth retardation, genital abnormalities, and ear abnormalities) syndrome (CS) was high on the differential diagnosis because of clinical concern for choanal atresia with bilateral dysmorphic microtia (Fig 1). However, significant and refractory hypocalcemia, lymphopenia, hypoplastic thymus, and undetectable TRECs led to consideration of 22q11.2 deletion syndrome (22q11.2DS, also known as DiGeorge syndrome, Shprintzen syndrome, conotruncal anomaly face syndrome, or velocardiofacial syndrome), with which there is significant phenotypic overlap with CS. (1)(2) The normal echocardiogram lowered suspicion

for 22q11.2DS, as congenital heart disease is present in up to 85% of those with the syndrome. (3) In addition, Kabuki syndrome, (4) diabetic embryopathy, (5) and embryopathy due to maternal retinoic acid exposure (6) were considered due to their phenotypic similarities to CS.

Nasal obstruction prompted consideration of congenital nasal pyriform aperture stenosis, which is critical to identify because of its association with holoprosencephaly. (7) The differential diagnosis for nasal obstruction also included choanal atresia, congenital nasal tumors, septal deviation, and congenital dacryocystoceles. The external ear deformities warranted consideration of branchio-oto-renal syndrome, renal coloboma syndrome, and mandibulofacial dysostosis with microcephaly, although notably, there is no known association between any of these conditions and hypocalcemia or lymphopenia. (8)(9)(10)

### Actual Diagnosis

Bilateral inner and middle ear dysplasia and bilateral membranous choanal atresia with associated posterior nasal aperture narrowing were identified on computed tomography of the head and face. There was no nasal pyriform aperture stenosis identified. Fundoscopy revealed a left chorioretinal coloboma and possible right optic nerve hypoplasia. Right-sided facial paralysis, consisting of absent right-sided facial activity during crying and attempted eye closure, was noted and consistent with right peripheral cranial nerve VII palsy. Subsequent brain magnetic resonance imaging redemonstrated choanal atresia with new findings of vermian hypoplasia with splaying of the cerebellar hemispheres, hypoplastic internal auditory canals, and inadequate visualization of cranial nerves VII and VIII (Fig 2). Renal involvement was excluded by urinalysis negative for proteinuria, normal renal and bladder ultrasonography findings, and normal blood pressure for age throughout admission. Review of maternal prenatal records and further history excluded the possibilities of maternal diabetes and maternal retinoic acid exposure.

In the setting of multiple major criteria for CS (choanal atresia, characteristic microtia with middle/inner ear anomalies, cranial nerve palsy, and coloboma), genetics was consulted and recommended performing karyotype, chromodomain helicase 7 (*CHD7*, on chromosome 8q12) mutation analysis, and microarray for further evaluation. These tests were performed simultaneously and revealed a normal karyotype and microarray with specific *CHD7* gene testing notable for a heterozygous known pathogenic variant for CS, c.7879 C>T, p.R2627X. (11) Up to 90% of patients with CS have mutations in the *CHD7*

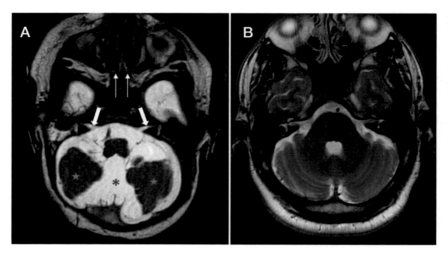

**Figure 2.** A. An axial T2-weighted magnetic resonance image at the level of the internal auditory canals demonstrates choanal atresia represented by soft tissue density completely effacing the bilateral choanae (thin arrows). The internal auditory canals are hypoplastic (thick arrows), with cranial nerves VII and VIII not visualized because of diminutive size. The cerebellar hemispheres (red stars) are splayed (ie, laterally displaced) in the setting of vermian hypoplasia. The blue asterisk represents the expected location of the normal vermis but contains only enlarged cerebrospinal fluid space because the cerebellar hemispheres do not fuse normally without a normal vermis. B. Comparative image of a different patient with normal structures.

gene. (12)(13)(14) Thus, the diagnosis of CS was confirmed based on these classic genotypic and phenotypic features.

## The Condition

CS is a rare genetic syndrome, with an incidence of approximately 1 in 10,000 to 15,000 live births. (15) Several proposed clinical criteria for the diagnosis of CS exist. (16)(17)(18) The lack of consensus guidelines is likely a reflection of the wide phenotypic spectrum of CS. Among all 3 sets of criteria, coloboma and choanal atresia are of major diagnostic significance. These guidelines differ in their inclusion of hypoplasia of the semicircular canals (17) and cranial nerve abnormalities (16) as major criteria (see Table 1 for a comparison of diagnostic guidelines). Notably, the absence of semicircular canals has been considered to be a hallmark feature of CS not typically associated with other syndromes. (14) All criteria necessitate the presence of at least 2 major criteria and some combination of minor criteria for diagnosis (Table 1). (16)(17)(18)

## Patient Course and Management

Pediatric otolaryngology performed endoscopic choanal atresia repair on day 6 after birth, and the patient was successfully extubated to room air immediately after the procedure. The infant had difficulty managing his secretions and poor oromotor coordination after extubation, requiring nasogastric tube feedings. Due to poor tolerance of feeds with gastroesophageal reflux, the infant ultimately required continuous feeds via a gastrostomy tube.

Profound, asymptomatic hypocalcemia was noted at 24 hours after birth and did not spontaneously improve on serial repeated measurements. In a healthy patient, hypocalcemia should stimulate the secretion of parathyroid hormone, which, in turn, acts on the bones to release calcium into the bloodstream and normalize serum calcium levels. However, this patient was found to have markedly low levels of intact parathyroid hormone, suggestive of inadequate parathyroid function consistent with primary hypoparathyroidism. Due to the severity of hypocalcemia with an inadequate response to intermittent intravenous boluses of calcium, the infant required a continuous calcium infusion for several days before transitioning to oral calcium repletion therapy.

In the setting of lymphopenia (defined as an absolute lymphocyte count $<1,800/\mu L$ [$<1.8 \times 10^9$/L] in the first year of life [1]), undetectable TRECs, and hypoplastic thymus on chest radiography, further studies were performed to characterize a potential immunodeficiency. T- and B-cell subsets, immunoglobulin (Ig) levels, and a lymphocyte enumeration panel were obtained (Table 2). Notable findings included low CD3+, CD3+CD4+, and CD3+/CD8+ T-cell subsets; elevated B-cell count; and low IgA, low-normal IgM, low IgE, and normal IgG levels. These results suggest an isolated T-cell deficiency. Although the IgM level was low, its presence suggests that B cells are functional, although it does not indicate whether class switching will occur. The normal level of IgG must be interpreted with caution because this is likely maternal in origin.

**Table 1.** Comparison of Major and Minor Diagnostic Criteria for CS and Clinical Diagnostic Criteria for CS

| BLAKE ET AL (16) | VERLOES (18) | HALE ET AL (17) |
|---|---|---|
| **Major Criteria** | | |
| Coloboma | Coloboma | Coloboma |
| Choanal atresia | Choanal atresia | Choanal atresia or cleft lip/palate |
| Characteristic ear abnormalities | Characteristic ear abnormalities (specifically hypoplastic semicircular canals) | Characteristic ear abnormalities |
| Cranial nerve dysfunction | | CHD7 pathogenic variant |
| **Minor Criteria** | | |
| Genital anomalies | Cranial nerve dysfunction | Cranial nerve dysfunction |
| Developmental delay | Characteristic ear abnormalities (specifically middle/external ear anomalies) | Developmental delay |
| Cardiovascular anomalies | Hypothalamo-hypophyseal dysfunction | Cardiovascular/esophageal anomalies |
| Growth retardation | Cardiovascular/esophageal malformations | Genital anomalies and hypothalamo-hypophyseal dysfunction |
| Cleft palate/lip | Intellectual disability | Feeding issues |
| Esophageal malformations (specifically tracheoesophageal fistula) | | Brain abnormalities |
| Characteristic facies | | Renal anomalies |
| | | Skeletal/limb anomalies |
| **Clinical Diagnostic Criteria** | | |
| All 4 major or 3 major plus 3 minor | Typical: 3 major or 2 major plus 2 minor | 2 major plus any number of minor |
| | Partial: 2 major plus 1 minor | |
| | Atypical: 2 major plus 0 minor or 1 major plus 3 minor | |

CS=CHARGE (coloboma, heart defects, atresia choanae, growth retardation, genital abnormalities, and ear abnormalities) syndrome.

Specialized flow cytometry studies were subsequently performed because severe combined immunodeficiency would require consideration of bone marrow transplant or thymic transplant. These studies confirmed that the T-cell numbers were below the tenth percentile for age. Reassuringly, the percentage of naive CD4 T cells was near normal, and the percentage of naive CD8 T cells was normal. Taken together, these findings suggest partial thymic hypoplasia rather than complete thymic aplasia. B-cell and natural killer cell populations were in the normal range on specialized flow cytometry. These findings again support the diagnosis of a T-cell immunodeficiency, which has been increasingly recognized in association with CS. (1)(19)(20) The effect of this T-cell immunodeficiency on humoral immunity will be elucidated on future laboratory studies with a lymphocyte stimulation panel and repeated immunoglobulin panels.

Because of his CD4 lymphocytopenia (lymphocyte count $<500/\mu L$ ($<0.50 \times 10^9$/L), prophylaxis for pneumocystis pneumonia with trimethoprim-sulfamethoxazole was initiated, any necessary blood products will be irradiated and cytomegalovirus negative, and live vaccines will be avoided.

Clinical Implications of Overlap Between CHARGE Syndrome and 22q11.2DS

Hypocalcemia and T-cell immunodeficiency are considered hallmark features of 22q11.2DS but are often overlooked features of CS. Not only are hypocalcemia and lymphopenia common in CS, they may be even more common in CS than in 22q11.2DS. (1) These overlapping phenotypic features are postulated to be secondary to the common genetic pathways involved in both syndromes. (1)(2)(19)(20)

**Table 2.** T and B Lymphocyte Subset Values

| CELL SUBSET | RESULTANT VALUE | REFERENCE RANGE |
|---|---|---|
| CD3, % | 13 | 60–85 |
| CD3 absolute count, cells/$\mu$L | 530 | 2300–7000 |
| CD19, % | 64 | 4–26 |
| CD19 absolute count, cells/$\mu$L | 2,549 | 600–1900 |
| CD3+CD4+, % | 11 | 41–68 |
| CD3+CD4+ absolute count, cells/$\mu$L | 442 | 1700–5300 |
| CD3+CD8+, % | 2 | 9–23 |
| CD3+CD8+ absolute count, cells/$\mu$L | 94 | 400–1700 |
| CD16+CD56+, % | 22 | 3–23 |
| CD16+CD56+ absolute count, cells/$\mu$L | 866 | 200–1400 |

In 22q11.2DS, the 40-gene deletion encompasses the *TBX1* gene, which is thought to be critical in the development of the hallmark features of the syndrome, as mutations in this gene alone result in a similar phenotype to 22q11.2DS. (21) The T-box transcription factor TBX1, encoded by the eponymous gene, regulates the expression of factors in downstream pathways involved in the genesis of the heart, thymus, parathyroid, and palate. (2)(21)(22) Much of the phenotype in 22q11.2DS is thought to result from the aberrant development of the third and fourth pharyngeal pouches, which eventually form the thymus and parathyroid gland. Thus, in 22q11.2DS, both lymphopenia and hypocalcemia are common due to the affected thymus and parathyroid.

In CS, the aberrant *CHD7* gene is postulated to regulate the transcription of the same end targets as the *TBX1* gene. (2) Thus, CS can be associated with immunodeficiency in the setting of thymic maldevelopment. (1)(19)(20) It has been previously observed that lymphopenia is tightly associated with hypocalcemia in patients with CS, which is hypothesized to result from similarly impaired development of the third and fourth pharyngeal pouches (and thus, the thymus and parathyroid gland) as is described in 22q11.2DS. (1) Our patient was found to have hypocalcemia and lymphopenia in the setting of hypoparathyroidism and partial thymic hypoplasia, further redemonstrating this association. Therefore, as has been previously proposed, we suggest universal screening of all patients with suspected CS and/or 22q11.2DS with a complete blood cell count with differential count, lymphocyte subset panel, and calcium level. (19)(20)

## Lessons for the Clinician

- The phenotypic features of 22q11.2 deletion syndrome and CHARGE syndrome (CS) are not mutually exclusive; thus, both should be considered in the setting of clinical concern for either condition.
- Hypocalcemia and immunodeficiency, particularly T-cell immunodeficiency, are frequently associated with CS.
- Complete blood cell count with differential count, lymphocyte subset panel, and calcium level should be routinely included in the laboratory evaluation for patients with suspected CS or 22q11.2 deletion syndrome.

## Acknowledgments

We thank Dr Min Hwang for her expert review of the manuscript. We extend special thanks to the family of this patient for their willingness to share and contribute to medical education through the publication of this case review.

The views expressed herein are those of the authors and do not reflect the official policy of the Department of the Army/Navy/Air Force, Department of Defense, or US Government.

*References for this article can be found at*
*https://doi.org/10.1542/pir.2020-003749.*

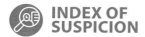

INDEX OF
SUSPICION

# Persistent Hypoxemia in an Asymptomatic 4-year-old Boy

Eliaz Brumer, MD,* David E. de Ángel Solá, MD,*† Mary-Jane Hogan, MD,‡ Laura Chen, MD*

*Department of Pediatrics, *Section of Respiratory, Allergy-Immunology, and Sleep Medicine and ‡Section of Hematology Oncology, Yale School of Medicine, New Haven, CT
†Department of Pediatrics, San Juan City Hospital, Río Piedras Medical Center, San Juan, Puerto Rico

## PRESENTATION

A 4-year-old boy with a history of anaphylaxis to peanuts and tree nuts presents to a local emergency department (ED) with an acute allergic reaction and a peripheral oxygen saturation by pulse oximetry ($SpO_2$) of 85% on room air. Before coming to the ED, he was in his usual state of health and playful. After eating a peanut, he developed acute facial swelling and pruritus, with no coughing or trouble breathing. In the ED he is afebrile with no signs of dyspnea, cyanosis, or respiratory distress. His pruritus and facial swelling improve after receiving intramuscular epinephrine and oral corticosteroids, which were given for potential anaphylaxis. Because he remains hypoxemic without respiratory complaints, he is transferred to our facility for further evaluation, where his heart rate and blood pressure are within normal limits for his age and his lungs are clear to auscultation bilaterally without wheezing. He has normal distal pulses, normal capillary refill, and no signs of digital clubbing or telangiectasias on his skin or oral mucosa. Administering supplemental oxygen results in $SpO_2$ less than or equal to 91%. His initial blood gas analysis on high-flow nasal cannula, 5 L/min of 100% oxygen, shows a $PaO_2$ of 410 mm Hg, with an alveolar-arterial (A-a) gradient of 254 mm Hg. Chest radiography reveals slight haziness on the right upper lobe but no signs of focal airspace disease, effusion, or pneumothorax. Due to persistent hypoxemia, he is admitted to the hospital for further evaluation and management.

A complete blood cell count shows mild normocytic normochromic anemia for his age (hemoglobin [Hb] level, 11.4 g/dL [114 g/L]), with normal methemoglobin levels and minimally elevated carboxyhemoglobin levels on co-oximetry. Blood testing reveals normal D-dimer and lactate dehydrogenase levels. Results of an Hb electrophoresis are normal. A 12-lead electrocardiogram and a transthoracic echocardiogram are normal. A noncontrast chest computed tomography (CT) scan shows saccular bronchiectasis in the apical segment of the right upper lobe associated with architectural distortion and atelectasis along the right major lung fissure. Ground-glass opacity is seen in the peripheral, anterior segment of the right upper lobe. Due to upper lobe findings on chest CT, a tuberculosis evaluation is performed. Results of the patient's purified protein derivative test and interferon-γ release assay are negative. Despite low $SpO_2$ levels, he continues to be playful and in no apparent respiratory distress on room air. After 9 days in the hospital, he is safely discharged with 2 L/min of supplemental oxygen and close outpatient follow-up.

AUTHOR DISCLOSER: Drs Brumer, de Ángel Solá, Hogan, and Chen have disclosed no financial relationships relevant to this article. This commentary does not contain a discussion of an unapproved/investigative use of a commercial product/device.

In the outpatient setting, his $Spo_2$ reading is 86% to 87% on room air, and he continues to be asymptomatic. A bubble echocardiogram shows no evidence of contrast on the left side either immediately or after 8 to 10 seconds. The pulmonologist, who sees him 14 days after discharge, places a saturation pulse oximetry probe on the fingers and earlobes of the patient's father and brother, who are found to also have similarly low peripheral oxygen saturations on room air despite no symptoms. Evaluation for a hemoglobinopathy by a hematologist shows a normal oxygen-Hb dissociation curve (performed by a reference laboratory compared with a control blood sample), and a genetic panel is sent for $\alpha$-, $\beta$-, and $\gamma$-globin gene mutations.

## DISCUSSION

### Differential Diagnosis

When assessing the causes of hypoxemia in children, one may consider the 5 most common causes, which consist of ventilation/perfusion (V/Q) mismatch, diffusion impairment, right-to-left shunt, hypoventilation, and low inspired $Po_2$. V/Q mismatch accounts for the most common causes of hypoxemia in children, (1) as is seen with pneumonia and lower airway obstruction (eg, asthma and bronchiolitis). The patient's chest radiograph and symptoms did not suggest pneumonia. Although he had symptoms of an acute allergic reaction, he showed no symptoms of upper or lower airway obstruction such as wheezing or stridor, and his ventilation was adequate and symmetrical. Although bronchiectasis could cause hypoxemia, especially with severe disease and during respiratory exacerbation, it mainly manifests with chronic productive cough and recurrent respiratory infections. (2) His chest CT scan also did not demonstrate signs of interstitial lung disease to suggest a diffusion limitation. His echocardiogram excluded a functional and anatomical cardiac cause of hypoxemia, and his bubble echocardiogram excluded most intrapulmonary and extrapulmonary shunt processes.

When persistent hypoxemia is present, an arterial blood gas analysis should be performed to calculate the A-a gradient to help elucidate the cause of hypoxemia of undetermined etiology. Normal $Pao_2$ is in the range of 80 to 100 mm Hg, (3)(4) and a normal A-a gradient in a healthy young individual is between 5 and 15 mm Hg. (5) A-a gradient increases with age secondary to changes in the structure and function of the respiratory system. A possibly helpful estimating formula of normal A-a gradient is (Age+10)/4. (6) An abnormally high A-a gradient suggests a diffusion limitation, V/Q mismatch, or a shunt, related to pathology in the alveolocapillary unit but will exclude hypoventilation (which

shows a normal gradient). Our patient had an initial abnormally elevated A-a gradient on 5 L/min of 100% oxygen, but this could have also been secondary to supplemental oxygen falsely heightening a relatively small baseline A-a gradient. When an arterial blood gas analysis was attempted on room air, the $Po_2$ was 77 mm Hg. A $Pao_2$ of 77 mm Hg (in a normal Hb) would correspond to an $Spo_2$ of 95% (3) (see the Table for reference values [3]), but our patient had a baseline $Spo_2$ in the mid-80%.

Several pathologic conditions, such as methemoglobinemia and carbon monoxide poisoning, may result in a reading of a falsely normal $Spo_2$ despite decreased oxygen-carrying capacity. (7)(8) Pulse oximetry determines $Spo_2$ by calculating the ratio between 2 pulsatile wavelengths of light (660 nm for oxygenated Hb and 940 nm for deoxygenated Hb) (9) transmitted through the cutaneous vascular bed. Although some Hb variants have true low oxygen affinities ($P50$) due to their structural mutations, with an equivalent low $Spo_2$, other hemoglobinopathies, such as Hb Lansing variant, cause falsely low saturation readings with normal oxygen affinities. (8)(10)(11)(12)(13) Different spectral properties of the Hb variants/pathologies may cause interference to pulse oximetry readings, showing unique absorbance patterns at 660 and 940 nm, resulting in true or falsely low $Spo_2$ levels. This should be a reminder of the limitations of common clinical tools and other factors affecting pulse oximetry performance. In patients who are clinically asymptomatic (as our patient) with a normal $Pao_2$, yet have a low $Spo_2$, Hb variant should be considered, even in the setting of normal Hb electrophoresis findings. Low $Spo_2$ in an asymptomatic biological parent and/or siblings may suggest a heritable hemoglobinopathy. A suggested approach to evaluating hypoxemia in children is included in the algorithm (Fig).

### The Condition

More than 1,000 hereditary hemoglobinopathies of the globin chains have been described, but only a small fraction of these mutations are associated with abnormal $Spo_2$ readings. (8) Extended gene analysis ultimately revealed that

**Table 1.** Correlation Between the Levels of Saturation of Peripheral Capillary Oxygen ($Spo_2$) and $Pao_2$ in Children with a Normal Oxyhemoglobin Dissociation Curve at a Temperature of 98.6°F (37°C) and pH of 7.4 (3)

| $Pao_2$ | $Spo_2$ |
|---|---|
| 40 mm Hg | 70% |
| 50 mm Hg | 80% |
| 60 mm Hg | 90% |
| 70 mm Hg | 95% |

the patient was heterozygous for Hb Lansing (*HBA2*:c.264C>G). This condition is associated with falsely low pulse oximeter readings with normal Pao$_2$ levels. (10)(11)(13)(14) Hb Lansing variant was first reported in 2 family members of Hispanic origin in 2009, (10) and it has been described in 8 other patients from 7 different families of Black, white, Mexican, Asian, and Omani descent. (7)(11)(12)(13)(14) Hb Lansing has a population frequency of 1 in 160,000. (15) It is caused by a CAC to CAG mutation at codon 87 of the alpha 2 gene, resulting in a histidine to glutamine substitution. (10)(11)(14)(15)

## Treatment/Management

Once Hb Lansing is confirmed, referral to genetics is recommended to determine whether other family members may also be affected. The cornerstone of management is reassurance and education to families of children affected by this condition. Obtaining baseline pulse oximeter readings

is important to determine typical Spo$_2$ ranges for these children because it may impact future medical management of breathing disorders. When there is concern for true hypoxemia, obtaining an arterial blood gas analysis to assess for Pao$_2$ is necessary. If the Pao$_2$ is normal, and/or there are no other causes of hypoxemia, oxygen treatment is not necessary. Notification of other health-care providers, including possible documentation such as a medical alert bracelet that patients can carry with them when seeing new providers, will be important to prevent unnecessary evaluation for asymptomatic hypoxemia in the future.

## Patient Course

After the diagnosis of Hb Lansing was made, the patient was taken off supplemental oxygen. His saturations during outpatient visits to his pulmonologist continue to range between 85% and 88% on room air. He continues to be

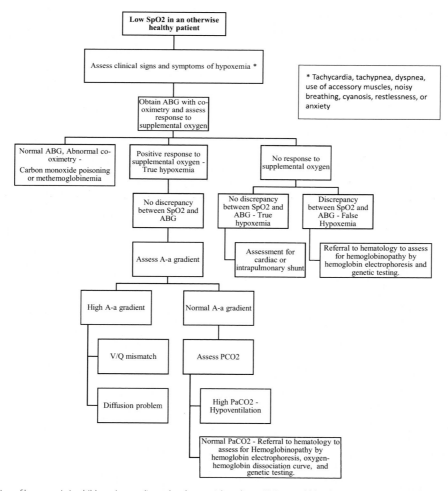

**Figure 1.** Evaluation of hypoxemia in children. A-a gradient, alveolar-arterial gradient; ABG, arterial blood gas; Spo$_2$, saturation of peripheral capillary oxygen; V/Q, ventilation/perfusion ratio.

asymptomatic and is growing well with no complaints. Repeated chest radiography performed to follow up on the area of bronchiectasis seen on previous chest CT showed resolution of the affected area and was normal. It is possible that the patient may have had traction bronchiectasis from atelectasis or another inflammatory or infectious process that concurrently occurred around the time of his admission. This finding was likely unrelated to his hemoglobinopathy variant.

## Lessons for the Clinician

- Most commonly, hypoxemia is secondary to cardiopulmonary diagnoses, where $Pao_2$ will correspond to an appropriate ($Spo_2$).

- If $Spo_2$ does not correspond to an appropriate $Pao_2$, clinicians should consider alternative, albeit rare, noncardiopulmonary diagnoses, including rare hemoglobinopathies, when unresolved hypoxemia is encountered.

- Education to patients and their family members about hemoglobinopathies that result in abnormal $Spo_2$ but normal $Pao_2$ is important to unnecessary medical investigations in the future and spare the families additional medical investigations and anxiety. (16)(17)

- We recommend an approach to evaluate hypoxemia in children as summarized in an algorithm (Fig 1).

*References for this article can be found at*
https://doi.org/10.1542/pir.2021-005293.

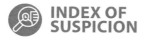

## INDEX OF SUSPICION

# Poor Growth in an 8-year-old Boy from Ethiopia

Jessica Hane, MD,* Cynthia Howard, MD, MPHTM,* Kelly Dietz, MD,† Stacene R. Maroushek, MD, PhD, MPH‡

*Division of Pediatric Hospital Medicine and
†Department of Radiology, Pediatrics Division, and
‡Division of Pediatric Infectious Disease, Hennepin Healthcare and University of Minnesota School of Medicine, Minneapolis, MN

## PRESENTATION

An 8-year-old boy presents to the adoption clinic for behavioral concerns and poor growth. The patient was adopted from Ethiopia 2 years before presentation. His medical history is significant for physical abuse and multiple housing transitions, including time spent in an orphanage. The patient does not have any immunization records but was noted to have a borderline Mantoux tuberculin skin test (TST) on arrival in the United States at an outside clinic. His parents are concerned that he has not grown taller since arriving in the United States. The patient has a good appetite and denies any fever, cough, or weight loss. He enjoys competitive running and has won multiple 5-km races.

In the clinic, the patient's weight is 48.7 lb (22.1 kg) (8th percentile on the Centers for Disease Control and Prevention [CDC] growth chart), height is 47.2 in (119.8 cm) (third percentile on the CDC growth chart), BMI is 15.4 (37th percentile on the CDC growth chart), and occipital frontal circumference is 21.3 in (54 cm) (75th percentile on the CDC growth chart). The physical examination reveals a small-for-age but otherwise well-appearing child. His lung fields are clear bilaterally, and no lymphadenopathy is appreciated. His complete blood cell count is normal except for a mildly elevated absolute eosinophil count of $600/\mu L$ ($0.6 \times 10^9/L$). His thyrotropin level is normal (1.61 mIU/L), free thyroxine level is normal (1.23 ng/dL [15.83 pmol/L]), insulinlike growth factor binding protein 3 level is normal (2,100 ng/mL [275 nmol/L]), insulinlike growth factor 1 level is low normal (63 ng/mL [8.25 nmol/L] (reference range, 62–349 ng/mL [8.12–45.72 nmol/L]), and 25-hydroxyvitamin D level is low normal (23 ng/mL [57.41 nmol/L]). Results of human immunodeficiency virus 1 and 2 antibody, hepatitis B surface antibody and antigen, hepatitis C antibody, and *Treponema pallidum* antibody tests are all negative. An interferon-γ release assay (IGRA) is positive, with a *Mycobacterium tuberculosis* antigen level of 5.55 IU/mL. A hand radiograph reveals a normal bone age. A chest radiograph from an outside clinic demonstrates possible left lung airspace disease. A follow-up chest computed tomographic (CT) scan performed with contrast demonstrates multiple prominent necrotic mediastinal and left hilar lymph nodes (Figs 1 and 2) as well as a small area of consolidation in the left lower lobe.

## DISCUSSION

### Diagnosis

The patient was admitted to the hospital for further evaluation and infectious disease consultation. The recommended evaluation included 3 induced sputum

AUTHOR DISCLOSURE Drs Hane, Howard, Dietz, and Maroushek have disclosed no financial relationships relevant to this article. This commentary does not contain a discussion of an unapproved/investigative use of a commercial product/device.

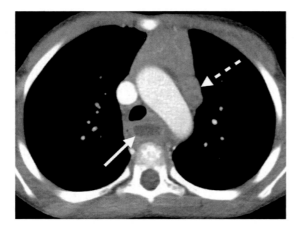

**Figure 1.** Axial contrast-enhanced computed tomographic scan through the mid-chest at the level of the aortic arch demonstrates an enlarged necrotic lymph node behind the trachea (solid arrow) and an enlarged partially necrotic prevascular lymph node (dashed arrow).

samples or gastric aspirates, ultrasonography-guided transesophageal biopsy of a mediastinal necrotic lymph node, stool ova and parasite examination, *Schistosoma* titers, and *Strongyloides* titers. The patient was unable to produce sputum for culture and, therefore, a nasogastric tube was placed to obtain 3 early-morning gastric aspirates. Three acid-fast bacillus stains and cultures were negative. Transesophageal biopsy of the left paratracheal lymph node revealed necrosis with acute and chronic inflammation and a rare granuloma with giant cells. Acid-fast bacillus stain and Grocott-Gömöri methenamine silver stain (used to identify *Pneumocystis jiroveci* and fungi) showed no mycobacterium, fungi, or pneumocystis, and the *M tuberculosis* immunoperoxidase stain was negative. Stool ova

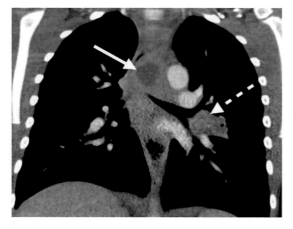

**Figure 2.** Coronal contrast-enhanced computed tomographic scan demonstrates the enlarged necrotic mediastinal lymph node (solid arrow) and an enlarged partially necrotic left hilar lymph node (dashed arrow).

and parasite examination revealed *Endolimax nana* and *Blastocystis hominis,* neither of which was felt to be a pathogen. *Schistosoma* IgG and *Strongyloides* IgG were negative.

Despite the negative culture results, pulmonary tuberculosis (TB) was diagnosed based on the patient's positive IGRA, CT findings of necrotic lymphadenopathy and nodular consolidation, and exposure history. In addition, his lymph node biopsy revealing rare granulomas with giant cells was suggestive of pulmonary TB.

The primary team also consulted endocrinology due to the patient's short stature and borderline low growth hormone studies. The endocrinology consultant concluded that his poor growth was likely secondary to untreated TB and recommended initiation of anti-TB treatment and a 3-month follow-up appointment in the endocrinology clinic.

The patient was started on isoniazid 300 mg orally daily (13 mg/kg per day), rifampin 450 mg orally daily (20 mg/kg per day), ethambutol 400 mg orally daily (20 mg/kg per day), and pyrazinamide 500 mg orally daily (20 mg/kg per day), as well as pyridoxine (vitamin $B_6$) 12.5 mg orally daily due to concerns about his nutritional status. He was discharged home with directly observed therapy administered by the Minnesota Department of Health through the local county health department. The patient had normal liver function tests before antituberculous therapy. After 2 weeks of treatment, his transaminase levels were elevated, with an aspartate aminotransferase level of 754 U/L (12.59 µkat/L) and an alanine aminotransferase level of 326 U/L (5.44 µkat/L). The 4-drug regimen was discontinued, and the drugs were individually restarted weekly. His transaminase levels returned to the normal range. He completed 2 months of the 4-drug regimen and an additional 4 months of isoniazid and rifampin without a recurrence of elevated transaminase levels.

### The Condition

*M tuberculosis* is a leading cause of morbidity and mortality worldwide but is rare in children in the United States. In 2018, only 9,029 cases of TB were reported in the United States, of which 372 (4.1%) were in children younger than 15 years. (1) Children account for approximately 11% of TB cases worldwide. (2) Accordingly, international adoptees have disproportionately high rates of TB and require prompt screening for TB on arrival in the United States. Children with a negative screen should be retested 3 to 6 months after arrival given the high proportion of initial false-negatives. (3)

The 2 types of screening tests for TB are the TST and the IGRA. The TST is recommended for children younger than 2 years, whereas the IGRA is recommended for children older than 2 years. (4)(5) BCG vaccination is not a contraindication to TST administration. (6) The TST and IGRA screening tests cannot distinguish between latent TB infection and active TB disease. Latent TB infection in children is defined by a positive immunologic screening test without physical findings or radiographic evidence of active TB. A chest radiograph is necessary if a child's screening test is positive or if they have signs and/or symptoms of TB. Chest radiographic findings of pulmonary TB include intrathoracic lymphadenopathy (best seen on the lateral view) and parenchymal opacities with or without cavitation (Ghon foci). (7)(8)

The clinical presentation of active TB in children is variable. Although some children are asymptomatic, others may progress to septic shock, multiorgan failure, and death. (6) Children younger than 2 years are more likely to have severe disease, school-age children are more likely to be asymptomatic, and adolescents typically present similarly to adults. (6) When present, the most common symptoms of pulmonary TB include cough, fever, chills, weight loss or poor weight gain, and linear growth delay. (5)

In children with symptoms of TB or abnormal imaging, the recommendation is to obtain sputum for staining and culture. For children who are unable to produce sputum, an early-morning gastric aspirate should be obtained via a nasogastric tube on 3 separate mornings. The diagnostic yield of induced sputum and gastric aspirates is low given that children commonly have paucibacillary disease. (9) Diagnosing active TB in children requires a high index of suspicion due to the challenges with laboratory testing. In the absence of culture data, the diagnosis of TB in

children is based on clinical signs and symptoms, a positive TST or IGRA, imaging consistent with TB disease, and exposure history. (5)(10)

In this case, the positive IGRA, the presence of granulomas on lymph node biopsy, and characteristic CT findings in a child adopted from a country with a high TB burden led us to the diagnosis of pulmonary TB.

## Management

Pediatric infectious disease consultation is recommended for patients with active TB. Empirical 4-drug treatment should be started while awaiting culture results. The first-line treatment for pulmonary TB is isoniazid 10 to 15 mg/kg per day, rifampin 15 to 20 mg/kg per day, pyrazinamide 30 to 40 mg/kg per day, and ethambutol 15 to 25 mg/kg per day. (5) For drug-susceptible *M tuberculosis*, the 4-drug regimen is recommended for 2 months, followed by an additional 4 months of isoniazid and rifampin. Pyridoxine supplementation is recommended for children with nutritional deficiencies or human immunodeficiency virus infection, pregnant adolescents, and exclusively breastfed infants. (5)(11) Treatment should be administered via directly observed therapy.

## Patient Course

The patient completed 2 months of 4-drug antituberculous treatment, followed by an additional 4 months of isoniazid and rifampin treatment. His weight and linear growth improved dramatically with treatment. His weight for age increased from the eighth percentile at his international adoption clinic visit to the 46th percentile just 6 months after completing antituberculous therapy (Fig 3A). Similarly, his stature for age increased from the fourth percentile to the 27th percentile in the same time frame (Fig 3B).

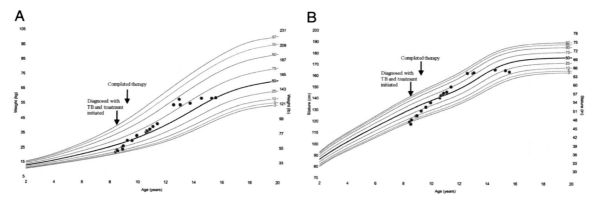

**Figure 3.** The patient's growth charts demonstrate a rapid increase in (A) weight for age and (B) stature for age after treatment of pulmonary tuberculosis. (Reprinted with permission from the Centers for Disease Control and Prevention, 2000.)

Because he had no immunization records, he received immunizations according to the CDC catch-up immunization schedule. The patient had a history of multiple adverse childhood experiences, including physical abuse and challenging transitions. He was referred to the Center for Neurobehavioral Development for further psychological evaluation and family resources.

Lessons for the Clinician
- *Mycobacterium tuberculosis* disproportionately affects foreign-born children from low- and middle-income countries, and prompt screening on arrival in the United States is essential. Repeated testing is recommended 3 to 6 months after arrival.
- Children with pulmonary tuberculosis (TB) are commonly asymptomatic but may present with cough, fever, chills, weight loss or poor weight gain, or isolated linear growth failure.
- Diagnosing active TB requires a high index of suspicion in children given the low yield of gastric aspirates and induced sputum.
- Active TB should be managed in consultation with pediatric infectious disease given the challenges in diagnosis, complicated medication regimen, and potential for medication toxicity.
- Internationally adopted children are often underimmunized, and it is important for clinicians to provide necessary catch-up immunizations on arrival in the United States.
- Pediatricians should provide resources and strategies for families to mitigate the effects of adverse childhood experiences on adopted children.

Acknowledgment
Thank you to Caitlin Bakker from the University of Minnesota for assisting with the literature review.

*References for this article can be found at*
https://doi.org/10.1542/pir.2020.001446

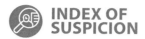

INDEX OF SUSPICION

# Preterm Infant with Severe Respiratory Distress and Intubation Difficulty

Atef Alshafei, MRCPCH,* Jamal Kassouma, MD,† Anwar Khan, MD,* Moustafa Hassan, MD*

*NICU, Pediatric Department, Dubai Hospital, Dubai, United Arab Emirates;
†ENT Department, Dubai Hospital, Dubai, United Arab Emirates

## PRESENTATION

A preterm male infant is born via cesarean delivery at 35 weeks of gestation with birth weight of 2.720 kg to a 30-year-old Gravida 3 Para 3 woman with an uneventful pregnancy, except for polyhydramnios. The infant is born nonvigorous, and T-piece positive pressure ventilation is given with improvement of the heart rate. The Apgar score is 5 and 7 at 1 and 5 minutes, respectively. He is noted to have severe respiratory distress and cyanosis, with oxygen saturations ranging from 54% to 60%, and intubation cannot be achieved even after several attempts using a small endotracheal tube of 2-mm internal diameter. Although the vocal cords are seen clearly, the endotracheal tube cannot be maneuvered beyond the cords. A nasopharyngeal tube is advanced and connected to noninvasive ventilation support with fraction of inspired oxygen of 1.0. The infant is admitted to the NICU and an on-call ear-nose-throat surgeon is urgently called. Upon examination, the infant is irritable and distressed with bilaterally decreased air entry and significant subcostal retractions. Heart examination reveals normal S1 and S2 heart sounds and grade II/VI systolic murmur over the left parasternal border. Abdominal examination is normal with bilaterally descended testes. At 30 minutes after birth, he is pink with saturation of 80% то 90%, but significant chest retractions and dysphonia are observed. Chest radiography shortly after birth reveals white-out lungs and abnormally dilated trachea (Fig 1). The ear-nose-throat surgeon places emergency tracheostomy tube 1 hour after birth, which is then connected to the mechanical ventilator (Fig 2). Surfactant is administered via tracheostomy tube, and saturation is maintained afterward. On day 2, he develops hypotension, with mean arterial blood pressure of 25 to 30 mm Hg and is transfused with packed red blood cells and inotropic support with dopamine and dobutamine is initiated. The initial sepsis screen is negative, and complete blood cell count is acceptable, except for hemoglobin of 8.9 gm/dL and hematocrit of 27.7%. Echocardiography reveals small apical ventricular septal defect measuring 1.4 mm. Brain and abdominal ultrasonography are normal. Karyotyping reveals the patient to be a normal 46XY male infant. One week after birth, he is referred to our unit for upper airway evaluation.

## DISCUSSION

### Differential Diagnosis

The unanticipated intubation difficulty in a newborn infant presenting with respiratory distress is a real challenge and could be due to the following:

AUTHOR DISCLOSURE Drs Alshafei, Kassouma, Khan, and Hassan have disclosed no financial relationships relevant to this article. This commentary does not contain a discussion of an unapproved/investigative use of a commercial product/device.

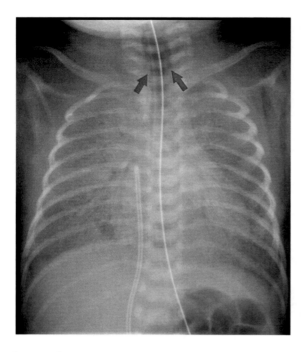

**Figure 1.** Chest radiograph on admission shows white out lungs and dilated trachea (red arrows).

-Congenital high airway obstruction syndrome (CHAOS): congenital subglottic stenosis (SGS), laryngeal and tracheal atresia, laryngeal web, and tracheal stenosis.

-Laryngeal cysts, subglottic hemangioma, and oropharyngeal or cervical tumors.

-Craniofacial abnormalities: Pierre Robin syndrome, Treacher Collins syndrome, and Goldenhar syndrome.

### Actual Diagnosis

Direct micro-laryngoscopy under general anesthesia reveals pinhole SGS grade IV (Video 1) (Fig 3). SGS is the third most common laryngeal anomaly after laryngomalacia and vocal cord palsy. (1) The incidence of congenital SGS is nearly 0.2% and represents ~5 to 10% of all SGS cases. (2)(3) The majority of SGS cases are acquired and occur secondary to prolonged intubation.

### THE CONDITION

Congenital SGS is defined as the narrowing of subglottic lumen to less than 4 mm in diameter in term infants and less than 3 mm in premature infants at the cricoid region with no previous history of intubation or trauma. (4) Congenital SGS is caused by developmentally small cricoid cartilage or thick submucosa secondary to recanalization failure in the subglottic area at the third month of gestation. (5) It is classified into 2 types: membranous the most common and cartilaginous. Some authors consider congenital SGS as a potential cause of CHAOS, although the cardinal diagnostic features are mainly prenatal ultrasound findings, (6) such as polyhydramnios, enlarged highly echogenic lungs, inverted hemidiaphragms, dilated trachea, and occasionally fetal

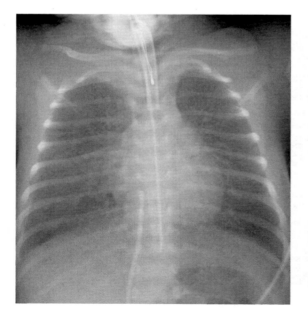

**Figure 2.** Chest radiograph after tracheotomy and surfactant replacement.

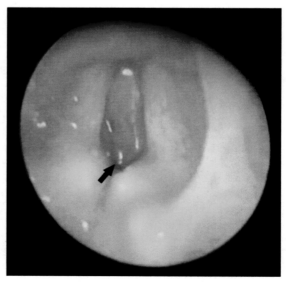

**Figure 3.** Grade IV congenital SGS as seen via direct laryngoscopy (black arrow).

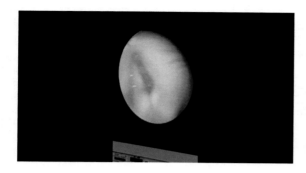

**Video 1.** Direct micro-laryngoscopy shows pinhole grade IV congenital SGS.

ascites. (7) The dilated tracheobronchial tree in severe forms of SGS may compress the esophagus resulting in polyhydramnios. These classical findings may not be collectively identified on prenatal ultrasound examination in cases of incomplete upper airway obstruction like in our case. Hence, the new definition of CHAOS includes any neonate who needs tracheotomy within 1 hour of birth, owing to severe upper airway obstruction, and cannot be directly intubated and ventilated through the trachea. (8) Despite the rarity and fatal outcomes of CHAOS, an early recognition before delivery may allow intrauterine intervention, namely, the ex utero intrapartum treatment. (9) During an ex utero intrapartum treatment procedure, an incision is made in the uterus during cesarean delivery allowing for partial delivery of the head and chest of the fetus while umbilical cord remains attached to the placenta. Then, direct laryngoscopy is done for evaluation of the upper airway and a tracheotomy is performed if severe obstruction is noted. Once the airway is secured, the umbilical cord is clamped, and the infant is handed over to the neonatologist for further resuscitation. SGS is graded according to the Myers-Cotton scale: grade I, up to 50% obstruction; grade II, 51% to 70%; grade III, 71% to 99%; and grade IV, no detectable lumen. (10) Grade IV congenital SGS is the most serious entity, owing to the early unexpected presentation of severe distress and dysphonia shortly after birth. Tracheostomy placement may be the life-saving procedure in this life-threatening event. Surprisingly, infants with grade III SGS may behave like those with milder forms of stenosis being completely asymptomatic for months and usually manifest as stridor with recurrent upper respiratory infections. Acquired SGS is more common than the congenital form and usually results from prolonged or repeated intubations with large or cuffed endotracheal tubes.

### Treatment and Management

SGS is typically diagnosed by direct laryngoscopy, although rigid bronchoscopy maybe needed to evaluate other associated congenital anomalies. The choice of therapy is individualized and depends on the clinical presentation and stridor severity. Many infants with mild-to-moderate SGS are conservatively managed with supportive care during exacerbations as most of them will outgrow the problem. However, severe cases presenting at birth or with significant stridor are initially managed by tracheotomy and may be corrected later by anterior cricoid split or reconstructive surgery and grafting.

### Patient Course

The patient is quickly weaned from ventilation and discharged from the hospital with the tracheostomy and planned full reconstructive surgery after 2 years. On the clinic follow-up after 6 months, he is thriving well and has normal developmental milestones for his age.

### Lessons for the Clinician

- High index of suspected congenital SGS should be considered in any infant with respiratory distress, absent or weak cry, and intubation difficulty at birth.
- An unanticipated intubation difficulty, although rare, requires a dedicated neonatal airway difficulty cart readily available at the labor suite and NICUs.
- Tracheotomy is a life-saving procedure offering the best chance of survival in severe cases of congenital SGS and CHAOS occurring at birth.

*References for this article can be found at*
*https://doi.org/10.1542/pir.2019-0028*

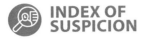

INDEX OF
SUSPICION

# Rapidly Progressive Respiratory Failure and Shock in a Healthy Teenager

Daniel Loeb, MD, MEd,* Kelli Paice, MD,† James Williams, MD,‡ Ranjit S. Chima, MD,* Andrew J. Lautz, MD*

*Division of Critical Care Medicine, Cincinnati Children's Hospital Medical Center, Department of Pediatrics, University of Cincinnati College of Medicine, Cincinnati, OH
†Division of Critical Care Medicine, Cincinnati Children's Hospital Medical Center, Cincinnati, OH
‡Division of Critical Care Medicine, University of Arkansas for Medical Sciences College of Medicine, Arkansas Children's Hospital

## PRESENTATION

A 14-year-old healthy girl is traveling from North Dakota to Kentucky on a family vacation. She lives on a farm, is a cross-country runner, and has had normal growth and development. Three days before presentation, she develops headaches, myalgias, fevers (101.3°F [38.5°C]), conjunctival injection, and fatigue. On the day of presentation, she develops dyspnea and cough, prompting her family to seek care.

In the emergency department, she has labored breathing but appears nontoxic. She is awake, conversant, and appropriate with a normal neurologic examination. She has tachycardia at 120 beats/min. Her blood pressure is 95/60 mm Hg, and her oxygen saturation ($Spo_2$) is 89% on room air. She has cold extremities but no rashes and delayed capillary refill with normal pulses. Her lungs are clear to auscultation bilaterally, and she has no murmur. Her abdominal examination is without hepatosplenomegaly and is soft.

Her initial labs are notable for a normal venous blood gas (pH 7.35, $Pco_2$ 35.0). Electrolytes are normal, with a blood urea nitrogen concentration of 10 mg/dL and creatinine concentration of 0.41 mg/dL. Alanine transaminase is 109 U/L (normal: <49.0 U/L), aspartate transaminase is 185 U/L (normal: 5–26 U/L), and procalcitonin is 1.09 ng/mL (normal: <0.1 ng/mL). The complete blood cell count is notable for polycythemia with a hemoglobin of 17.4 gm/dL (normal: 12.0–16.0 gm/dL) and leukopenia with a white blood cell count of $3.86 \times 10^3/\mu L$ (normal: $4.50–11.0 \times 10^3/\mu L$) with 82% segmented neutrophils, 10% band cells, and 8% monocytes.

She is started on a bolus of normal saline and is placed on oxygen via a nasal cannula. However, the fluid bolus is stopped because of worsening hypoxemia, prompting escalation to a nonrebreather. A chest radiograph is performed (Fig 1), and she is given ceftriaxone and is admitted to the PICU.

Once in the PICU, she is placed on positive pressure ventilation via a nasal mask with adequate oxygenation. Her heart rate remains mildly tachycardic, but her blood pressure is normotensive; however, her extremities remain cool. She is placed on maintenance intravenous fluids.

Twelve hours after arrival to the ICU, her respiratory status rapidly deteriorates, with a $Spo_2$ of 92% on 100% fraction of inspired oxygen ($Fio_2$). She develops worsening shock during this time frame, as evidenced by a mixed venous saturation decreasing from 70% to 42% and lactate increasing from 2.2 to 7.67 mmol/L (normal: 0.70–2.10 mmol/L). An echocardiogram test result reveals mildly diminished left ventricular function with a moderate pericardial effusion without tamponade

**AUTHOR DISCLOSURE:** Drs Loeb, Paice, Williams, Chima, and Lautz have disclosed no financial relationships relevant to this article. This commentary does not contain a discussion of an unapproved/investigative use of a commercial product/device.

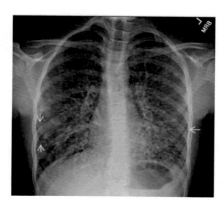

**Figure 1.** Initial chest radiograph in the emergency department. This film reveals noncardiogenic pulmonary edema with trace fluid in the fissures (yellow arrows).

physiology. A second chest radiograph is performed (Fig 2). She is intubated but unable to achieve a blood $SpO_2$ greater than 80% despite high ventilator settings. Her oxygen saturation index (OSI) 1 hour after intubation is 25 (using a mean airway pressure of 18 cm $H_2O$ on 100% $FIO_2$ with $SpO_2$ of 70%), prompting an extracorporeal membrane oxygenation (ECMO) evaluation.

She develops hypotension requiring frequent fluid boluses, in addition to vasopressin and epinephrine infusions. The decision is made to cannulate her to venous-arterial ECMO (VA-ECMO). During cannulation, ~24 hours after presentation and 2 hours after intubation, her OSI continues to deteriorate, reaching 80 (mean airway pressure of 52 cm $H_2O$ on 100% $FIO_2$ with $SpO_2$ of 60%) and resulting in a 9-minute cardiac arrest. She receives high-quality cardiopulmonary resuscitation, resulting in the return of spontaneous circulation. Shortly after spontaneous circulation returns, a VA-ECMO is successfully initiated.

## DISCUSSION

### Differential Diagnosis

Pediatric acute respiratory distress syndrome (pARDS) is defined as hypoxemia: 1) occurring within 7 days of a clinical insult, 2) exempting cardiac failure or fluid overload, and 3) demonstrating chest imaging findings of a new infiltrate/s consistent with acute parenchymal lung disease. (1) The severity of pARDS is stratified by oxygen support requirement, expressed as an $SpO_2/FIO_2$ ratio before mechanical ventilation and either an oxygenation index (OI) or OSI after intubation. Severe pARDS is defined as an OSI of equal to or greater than 12.3 (or an OI of 16), with the transfer to an ECMO center recommended when the OSI is greater than 32.5 (or OI >25). (2) The most common cause of pARDS is primary lung disease (eg, pneumonia), followed by sepsis and, much less frequently, trauma. (3) Cold shock, which may represent a vascular compensatory response to poor cardiac output but can also reflect a response to profound intravascular volume depletion, manifests owing to high systemic vascular resistance and features cold extremities, weak pulses, and delayed cap refill. The non-pARDS causes of respiratory failure are many and include neurologically mediated inadequate respiratory drive, upper airway obstruction, cardiogenic-pulmonary edema, and neuromuscular weakness.

Worsening hypoxemia and radiographic findings concerning for lung disease should prompt clinicians to think about pARDS and then treat accordingly. Most children who have pARDS have an acute infectious process; therefore, prompt antibiotic administration is key to improving mortality in these patients, along with appropriate ventilator treatment. (4) In this patient, blood, urine, and bronchoalveolar lavage bacterial culture results were all negative. Polymerase chain reaction test results for multiple common

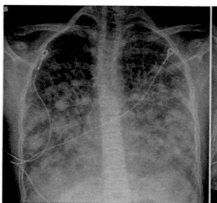
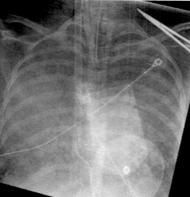

**Figure 2.** Rapid progression of pulmonary edema and pleural effusions. The patient was intubated and cannulated onto VA-ECMO in the interim between the two radiographs, which were taken ~6 hours apart.

viruses, including SARS-CoV-2, were also negative. Her mildly diminished cardiac function alone did not explain the severity and rapid progression of her respiratory failure.

## Actual Diagnosis

Although results were not available until well after her presentation, serology diagnostics revealed hantavirus-positive immunoglobin M and immunoglobin G. A wide array of laboratory results and studies to look for alternative diagnoses were completed as well. Ultimately, no other viral, bacterial, or fungal study results were positive. An immune dysregulation evaluation result was also negative. After cannulation to VA-ECMO, the patient remained in cardiorespiratory failure for several days and required continuous renal replacement therapy for anuria and 16% fluid overload (weight was up 7 kg from admission). Four days after initiation of ECMO, her lung compliance, pulmonary edema, and effusions improved (Fig 3). The ECMO was weaned, and she was decannulated 6 days after presentation. She was extubated on hospital day 13, began making urine on day 16, and was liberated from dialysis on day 20. She was discharged from the hospital at her neurologic baseline with no functional deficits.

## The Condition

Hantavirus (also called orthohantavirus) comprises a genus of negative-sense RNA viruses that are typically carried by rodents. (5) Although it does not cause symptomatic infection in rodents, hantavirus is the causative agent of both hantavirus hemorrhagic fever with renal syndrome (HFRS) and hantavirus pulmonary syndrome (HPS) in humans, who serve as accidental hosts. (6) First described in 1951 along the Hantan River in South Korea (from which the virus gets its name), hantavirus was presumed to be responsible for

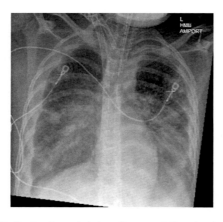

**Figure 3.** Chest radiograph 4 days after presentation, showing improvement in bilateral edema and pleural effusions.

~3,000 cases of shock associated with renal failure among US soldiers during the Korean War. (7) There are many variants of hantavirus globally, with native variants in both North and South America, as well as Asia and Europe. (8) In the United States, the vast majority of cases occur west of the Mississippi River. (9) A thorough travel history is needed to assess risk of exposure because the incubation period can allow some distance from point of transmission in an endemic area. Person-to-person transmission is rare but has been reported with a specific viral strain in South America. (10) Diagnosis of hantavirus is confirmed by at least one of the following findings: 1) a positive serological test result, 2) evidence of a viral antigen, or 3) the presence of amplifiable RNA sequences in either blood or tissue. (11)

Classically, HFRS and HPS are thought of as separate syndromes, with HFRS typically presenting in Asia and HPS presenting in the Americas. However, there is a great deal of overlap between the two, owing to a shared pathophysiology. (12) After inhalation of the virus from rodent excrement, the virus invades via alveolar macrophages in the lungs. From there, the virus causes severe breakdown of endothelial integrity in both the lungs and the kidneys, resulting in the profound kidney and lung injury seen in HFRS and HPS, respectively. (13)

Symptomatic HFRS occurs after a 1 to 6 week incubation period and carries ~12% mortality risk. (8)(14) Early disease is characterized by several days of flu-like symptoms, which consist of fevers, myalgias, and malaise. Petechiae and conjunctival injection can also be seen during this early phase. (15) Subsequently, profound capillary leak develops, which results in hypotension and shock. The degree of pulmonary involvement in HFRS is variable, albeit less than in HPS. Patients who have HFRS display a variety of kidney injury, resulting in oliguria that requires dialysis. Most patients are liberated from dialysis as they convalesce. (6)

Symptomatic HPS occurs after a 1- to 5-week incubation period. (16) Since 1993, 833 diagnoses of hantavirus have been given in the United States with 94% occurring west of the Mississippi River. Of the 833 cases, 35% of patients died. (9) The prodrome of HPS is like that of HFRS, with several days of fever, myalgias, and headache. Subsequently, hyperacute noncardiac pulmonary edema develops, which is associated with worsening hemoconcentration as the pulmonary endothelium fails and intravascular volume leaks into the lungs. (10) The disease peaks at ~5 to 7 days, but acute renal failure and respiratory failure secondary to shock can persist.

## Treatment and Management

Hantavirus, whether HFRS or HPS, is a self-limiting condition with spontaneous resolution occurring 1 to 2 weeks after the onset of severe symptoms. There is no specific treatment for hantavirus infection other than supportive care. Although hantavirus has been well-described west of the Mississippi River, this case occurred 400 miles east of the Mississippi River, which is exceedingly rare but was explained by her travel history.

The most important complications of hantavirus infection are acute respiratory failure, shock, and acute renal failure. Given the severity of the illness, hantavirus infections often require intubation, vasoactive support, dialysis, and sometimes ECMO. The mortality for HFRS and HPS are both high; therefore, patients at reasonable risk of hantavirus infection should be monitored closely during the early phases of illness for acute decompensation at a center that can treat complications from the disease. The severe pulmonary vascular leak from a hantavirus infection results in profound intravascular hypovolemia. Fluid resuscitation should be equally aggressive during the escalating phase of the disease. Pediatric intensivists should be prepared to treat severe and hyperacute respiratory failure.

Despite her 9-minute cardiac arrest and VA-ECMO course, the patient did well after disease convalescence, and she was ultimately discharged from the hospital without requiring supplemental oxygen or dialysis. She continues to thrive and, on her subsequent follow-up, has no lasting sequelae of hantavirus. Her renal function has returned to normal, and her lungs have healed. She has returned to school full-time, is enrolled in regular class, and exercises daily.

Lessons for the Clinician
- Hantavirus is a rare but rapidly progressive cause of acute respiratory failure and shock in both children and adults.
- Hantavirus occurs primarily in the western half of the United States and Asia, after exposure to rodent excrement, and can have an incubation period lasting up to 6 to 8 weeks.
- Patients who have HPS or HFRS require supportive treatment for respiratory distress syndrome, shock with profound capillary leak, and renal failure. No specific treatment for hantavirus exists.
- Cold extremities, delay cap refill, and other signs of cold shock in addition to a rising hematocrit all indicate worsening capillary leak and hemoconcentration and portend the imminent acute pulmonary phase of illness.

*References for this article can be found at*
*https://doi.org/10.1542/pir.2022-005807*

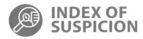

INDEX OF
SUSPICION

# Refractory Pneumonia in a 12-year-old Girl with Hemoglobin SS Disease

Violeta G. Tregoning, DO,* Krista Parran, MD,* Ashleigh S. Watson, MD,* Michelle L. Mitchell, MD*

*Medical College of Wisconsin and Children's Wisconsin, Milwaukee, WI

## PRESENTATION

A 12-year-old girl with hemoglobin SS disease presents with fever, cough with sputum production, chest pain, right shoulder pain, bilateral leg pain and decreased appetite before the coronavirus disease 2019 pandemic. She had a 2-day admission 1 week earlier for acute chest syndrome, her second hospitalization in 12 months. She received intravenous (IV) ceftriaxone and azithromycin but no blood products and was discharged on 5 more days of amoxicillin and 3 more days of azithromycin after resolution of her symptoms of fever, cough, chest pain, right shoulder pain, and decreased appetite. She now reports that her symptoms have been persistent since this most recent discharge despite the antibiotic treatment. The cough has been worsening, and the bilateral leg pain is new compared with her symptoms during the most recent hospitalization. She denies vomiting, diarrhea, abdominal pain, rashes, headache, or vision changes. It is influenza season, but she has no known sick contacts and no exposures to zoonotic hosts, and she lives in an urban area in the northern Midwest.

Vital signs include a temperature of 102.9°F (39.4°C), heart rate of 148 beats/min, blood pressure of 121/69 mm Hg, respiratory rate of 28 breaths/min, and oxygen saturation of 98% on room air. Physical examination shows an alert but uncomfortable-appearing girl with reproducible pain on palpation of her sternum, rib cage, and right shoulder. Her lung examination reveals diminished breath sounds over the right middle lobe but is otherwise clear to auscultation. Cardiac and abdominal examination findings are normal. There is no scleral icterus or jaundice. A normal saline bolus is given, as is morphine and ketorolac for pain control. Her chest radiograph shows worsening consolidation of the medial basal segment of the right lower lobe (Fig 1) compared with the imaging during her previous hospitalization. Initial laboratory data show the following: white blood cell count, 22,200/μL ($22.2 \times 10^9$/L) (reference range, 4,000–15,300/μL [$4.0$–$15.3 \times 10^9$/L]), which is elevated compared with her baseline and most recent hospitalization values; hemoglobin level, 10.9 g/dL (109 g/L) (reference range, 12.0–15.0 g/dL [120–150 g/L]) but within her baseline range of 10 to 12 g/dL (100-120 g/L) and unchanged from previous hospitalization values; reticulocyte percentage, 4.2% (reference range, 0.5%–2.2%); and platelet count, $429 \times 10^3$/μL ($429 \times 10^9$/L) (reference range, $150$–$450 \times 10^3$/μL [$150$–$450 \times 10^9$/L]). A blood culture sample is collected. Empirical ceftriaxone and azithromycin are started, and the patient is admitted to the hospital acute care floor for further management.

**AUTHOR DISCLOSURE:** Drs Tregoning, Parran, Watson, and Mitchell have disclosed no financial relationships relevant to this article. This commentary does not contain a discussion of an unapproved/investigative use of a commercial product/device.

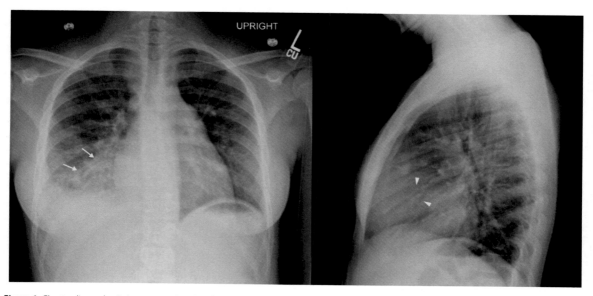

**Figure 1.** Chest radiographs. A. Anteroposterior view showing consolidation of the medial basal segment of the right lower lobe (arrows). B. Lateral view showing a focal airspace opacity in the anterior right middle lung (arrowheads). (Courtesy of Children's Wisconsin Radiology Department [Pooja Thakrar, MD].)

Despite 3 days of empirical antibiotic treatment, daily fevers persist. Repeated and additional laboratory tests show a white blood cell count of 35,160/μL (35.16 × 10⁹/L), with 82.7% neutrophils (reference range, 36%–72%); a platelet count of 1,889 × 10³/μL (1,889 × 10⁹/L); an erythrocyte sedimentation rate of 125 mm/hr (reference range, 0–10 mm/hr); a C-reactive protein level of 25.5 mg/dL (255 mg/L) (reference range, 0–1 mg/dL [0–10 mg/L]); a procalcitonin level of 52 ng/dL (0.52 μg/L) (reference range, <11 ng/dL [<0.11 μg/L]); a uric acid level of 1.6 mg/dL (0.10 mmol/L) (reference range, 2.0–6.3 mg/dL [0.12–0.37 mmol/L]); a lactate dehydrogenase level of 425 U/L (7.10 μkat/L) (reference range, 370–840 U/L [6.18–14.03 μkat/L]); and an angiotensin-converting enzyme inhibitor level of 29.0 U/L (483.3 nkat/L) (reference range, 13–100 U/L [216.7–1,666.7 nkat/L]). Several blood culture samples have been collected and continue to be without growth. Additional testing, including Epstein-Barr virus and cytomegalovirus serologies and nucleic acid amplification testing for enteric pathogens, parvovirus B19, influenza A and B, adenovirus, parainfluenza, mycoplasma, and *Chlamydia pneumoniae*, are sent to the laboratory. Urine *Blastomyces* and *Histoplasma* antigens are also collected.

A computed tomographic scan of the chest with contrast shows a masslike consolidation in the right lower lobe, scattered bilateral pulmonary nodules, subcarinal and right hilar lymphadenopathy, and a small right pleural effusion (Fig 2). A magnetic resonance image of the

shoulder shows no evidence of osteomyelitis, but multiple slightly enlarged lymph nodes are incidentally noted in the right axillary and lower cervical chain region. Antibiotic therapy is empirically broadened to cefepime and linezolid; however, the patient continues to have daily fevers.

A bronchoscopy with a bronchoalveolar lavage (BAL) reveals a mucus plug in a subsegmental bronchus branching from the right lower lobe bronchus. BAL fluid is sent for analysis, Gram-stain, and aerobic, anaerobic, mycobacterial, fungal, and viral cultures.

## DIFFERENTIAL DIAGNOSIS

Acute chest syndrome can be caused by pulmonary infarction, fat embolism, or, most commonly, viral or bacterial pathogens. The most common bacterial pathogens are *Streptococcus pneumoniae*, *Staphylococcus aureus*, and atypical pathogens such as *Chlamydia* and *Mycoplasma*. Viral pneumonia was initially considered, but the pattern of focal consolidation on chest radiograph in combination with persistent fevers, elevated inflammatory markers, and negative viral studies made this diagnosis less likely. This patient was treated for community-acquired pneumonia, but she continued to worsen. The differential diagnosis was broadened to include less common pathogens such as fungi, postobstructive pneumonia due to congenital airway malformation, extraluminal airway compression, neoplasm, and pulmonary sarcoidosis. Bronchoscopy was performed to evaluate for an airway malformation or obstruction and to try to isolate an infectious

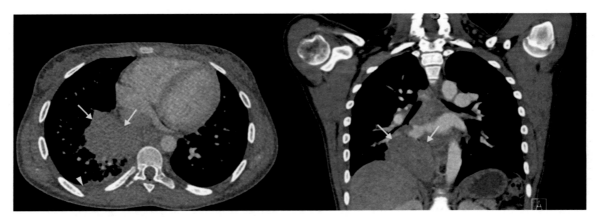

**Figure 2.** Chest computed tomographic scans with contrast. Coronal (A) and axial (B) views showing a mass-like consolidation in the right lower lobe (arrows) and a small right pleural effusion (arrowhead). (Courtesy of Children's Wisconsin Radiology Department [Pooja Thakrar, MD].)

organism. Sarcoidosis was considered, but her young age, acute onset, chest radiography pattern, lack of extrapulmonary disease, and normal angiotensin-converting enzyme inhibitor level made this etiology less likely.

## ACTUAL DIAGNOSIS

BAL direct examination shows broad-based budding yeasts, and culture speciates into *Blastomyces dermatitidis*, revealing the diagnosis. Urine antigens for *Blastomyces* and *Histoplasma* are positive. Viral and atypical bacterial testing results are negative. The patient is started on amphotericin, and oral itraconazole and antibacterials are discontinued. A full-body and brain magnetic resonance image reveals no extrapulmonary fungal infection. Inflammatory markers and thrombocytosis decrease after initiation of antifungal treatment.

## DISCUSSION

*B dermatitidis* and *Blastomyces gilchristii* are 2 species of dimorphic fungi endemic to North America, predominantly in the Great Lakes region, the Mississippi and Ohio river valleys, and the St Lawrence River areas. They are dimorphic fungi and thrive in forested, acidic, sandy soils near water containing decaying vegetation or organic matter. When spores of either species are inhaled, they can give rise to a systemic pyogranulomatous infection called *blastomycosis*. Acute pulmonary blastomycosis is 1 manifestation of the infection. Incubation time after environmental exposure to the spores is generally 3 to 6 weeks. Presenting symptoms can include any combination of the following: cough, fever, shortness of breath, weight loss, night sweats, chills, hemoptysis, and pleuritic chest pain. (1) Acute pulmonary

blastomycosis is frequently indistinguishable from bacterial or viral pneumonia by history and physical examination findings. (2) Blastomycosis can also cause a chronic pneumonia presenting as low-grade fevers, productive cough, hemoptysis, chest pain, and weight loss. Pulmonary blastomycosis can progress to disseminated blastomycosis, affecting the skin as verrucous lesions or nodules; the musculoskeletal system as osteomyelitis or arthritis; the genitourinary system as prostatitis, epididymo-orchitis, or tubo-ovarian abscess; or the central nervous system (CNS) as meningitis, epidural, or intracranial abscesses. However, some patients may develop the aforementioned extrapulmonary manifestations without preceding symptomatic *Blastomyces* pneumonia. (3)

Chest radiographs in pulmonary blastomycosis most often show alveolar infiltrates. These are more often unilateral and in the lower lobes but can also involve multiple lobes, including upper lobes. Chest radiographs can also show a reticulonodular patterns or can be without airspace consolidation. (4) Computed tomographic scans can show nodules, consolidations without cavitation, or tree-in-bud opacities (areas of centrilobular nodules with a linear branching pattern that can be seen in bacterial or fungal pneumonia, cystic fibrosis, bronchiolitis, and neoplasms). (5)

Definitive diagnosis is established by growth of organism from culture or by visualization of organism on tissue histologic analysis. Colonization with blastomycosis has not been reported in the literature. Cultures of the mold on Sabouraud dextrose agar grow in 1 to 4 weeks, with BAL samples yielding a positive culture in approximately 92% of patients. Cytologic examination of sputum, pleural fluid, or BAL fluid has low diagnostic yield but is available in shorter time courses than culture. If present, *Blastomyces* cells are easily differentiated from other fungal cells based on size and characteristic morphology of the broad-based budding yeast. (6) Serologic testing can be useful but often cross-reacts with other mycoses, especially *Histoplasma*. Likewise, antigen testing cross-reacts with other mycoses, but sensitivity of urine antigen testing for mycoses is good. (1) Antigen levels can also be useful in monitoring disease course, as levels decline with successful treatment and increase with disease recurrence. (7) A thorough history and physical examination should be conducted with possible extrapulmonary manifestations in mind. Further targeted or whole-body imaging may be needed depending on the presentation.

## Management

The choice and duration of treatment of blastomycosis depends on several factors, including clinical form, severity of disease, and immune status. In severe or disseminated disease, including extrapulmonary or progressive pulmonary disease and in patients who are immunocompromised, a lipid formulation of amphotericin B or amphotericin B deoxycholate (conventional amphotericin formulations) should be initiated. (8) Amphotericin B deoxycholate is associated with higher toxicity risk compared with the lipid formulation. The adverse effects associated with amphotericin B include nephrotoxicity, fever, rigors, nausea, and vomiting. In CNS infection, the lipid formulation of amphotericin B is preferred because of fewer adverse effects and possibly improved CNS penetration. (7) Therapy can transition to oral agents (itraconazole or voriconazole) once there is improvement in symptoms (fever, cough, night sweats, muscle pain, chest pain, and fatigue), which is usually seen after 1 to 2 weeks from initiation of IV treatment for mild or moderate disease and after 4 to 6 weeks for CNS or severe disease.

The Infectious Diseases Society of America has published clinical practice guidelines for the management of blastomycosis, with therapeutic strategy partially based on disease severity (mild, moderate, or severe) but without clearly defining each severity level. Consultation with an infectious disease physician or other provider with experience in the management of blastomycosis is recommended. Oral therapy in mild or moderate disease is most commonly itraconazole, although voriconazole has been a successful alternative treatment for *Blastomyces* CNS disease, refractory blastomycosis, and immunosuppressed

patients. (8) Both posaconazole and isavuconazole have also been proved effective and are becoming more popular alternative treatments. Additional alternative treatments for mild to moderate disease can consist of fluconazole or ketoconazole; however, these are less effective compared with itraconazole. Duration of oral therapy should generally be 6 to 12 months after 1 to 2 weeks of IV therapy in mild or moderate disease, at least 12 months for osteoarticular infections, and at least 12 months after 4 to 6 weeks of IV therapy in severe or CNS disease.

## Patient Course

Amphotericin is discontinued on day 10 of antifungal treatment (hospital day 18) once the patient is afebrile for 48 hours, her oral itraconazole serum level is therapeutic, and she has improvement in all her presenting symptoms. She is discharged from the hospital on day 22 of her current hospitalization and continues single therapy with oral itraconazole for 12 months with good adherence. Chest radiography findings returned to baseline by 3 months of treatment.

## Lessons for the Clinician

- Blastomycosis or other endemic fungus must be considered on the differential diagnosis in patients with suspected pneumonia not responding to conventional treatment, especially in those who live or have recently traveled in endemic areas.
- Acute pulmonary blastomycosis presents variably with cough, fever, shortness of breath, chest pain, and/or productive cough and may also include weight loss, hemoptysis, and night sweats as presenting symptoms.
- Diagnosis is made by culture of bronchoalveolar lavage washings, sputum, or pleural fluid or by histologic analysis of tissue specimens. Serum and urine antigens are noninvasive tests to help guide further diagnostic testing or otherwise support a clinical diagnosis.
- Patients diagnosed as having pulmonary blastomycosis must be evaluated for extrapulmonary disease to determine treatment agent and duration.

*References for this article can be found at*
https://doi.org/10.1542/pir.2020-003475.

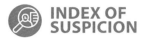

## INDEX OF SUSPICION

# Respiratory Distress and Macular Rash in a 13-year-old Girl

Courtney Pette, BS,* Giancarlo Toledanes, DO,† Maria Pereira, MD‡

*Baylor College of Medicine, Houston, TX
†Division of Pediatric Hospital Medicine and
‡Division of Rheumatology, Department of Pediatrics, Texas Children's Hospital, Baylor College of Medicine, Houston, TX

## PRESENTATION

A previously healthy 13-year-old girl presents with 7 days of fever, congestion, and cough. Five days before presentation she was seen by her primary care physician and diagnosed clinically as having community-acquired pneumonia and started on amoxicillin. Because of continued fevers, her primary care physician changed her antibiotic to cefdinir after 3 days. She presented to the emergency department 2 days later with dyspnea and worsening cough. She had no other preceding illness or sick contacts.

On presentation she is afebrile and vital signs include a heart rate of 136 beats/min, a respiratory rate of 56 breaths/min, and oxygen saturation of 87% on room air. Her growth chart demonstrates weight and length below the third percentile for age with no recent weight loss. The physical examination is significant for a thin female with pallor, dry mucous membranes, pale conjunctivae, dyspnea with bilateral decreased breath sounds and diffuse crackles, and nonblanching, nontender erythematous macules consistent with nonpalpable purpura and petechiae on the lower legs, forearms, and palmar aspect of hands bilaterally (Fig 1). Laboratory values demonstrate a hemoglobin level of 8.7 g/dL (87 g/L), a white blood cell count of 11,500/μL (11.5×10⁹/L), a platelet count of 314×10³/μL (314×10⁹/L), an erythrocyte sedimentation rate of 90 mm/hr (reference range, <20 mm/hr), a C-reactive protein level of 35 mg/dL (350 mg/L; reference range,<1 mg/dL [<10 mg/L]), a prothrombin time of 18.2 seconds (reference range, 10.5–15.7 seconds), a fibrinogen level of 650 mg/dL (19.11 g/L; reference range, 220–440 mg/dL [6.47–12.94 g/L]), and a D-dimer level of 8.6 μg/mL (47.09 nmol/L; reference range, <0.4 μg/mL [<2.19 nmol/L]). Urine microscopy is positive for 5 to 10 red blood cells and no protein. A chest radiograph reveals bilateral diffuse opacities (Fig 2). Computed tomography of the chest shows air space consolidation with superimposed reticular and ground glass opacities (Fig 3). She is admitted to the hospital on a high-flow nasal cannula and is treated empirically with vancomycin, ceftriaxone, and azithromycin for suspected bacterial sepsis and community-acquired pneumonia that is unresponsive to oral antibiotics.

She requires increasing respiratory support to 12 L/min and a fraction of inspired oxygen of 60%. A repeated complete blood cell count 2 days later demonstrates severe normocytic anemia with a hemoglobin level of 6.3 g/dL (63 g/L)

AUTHOR DISCLOSURE: Ms Pette and Drs Toledanes and Pereira have disclosed no financial relationships relevant to this article. This commentary does not contain a discussion of an unapproved/investigative use of a commercial product/device.

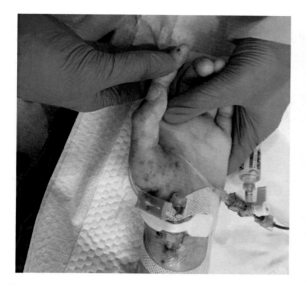

**Figure 1.** Purpuric and petechial rash on the hand.

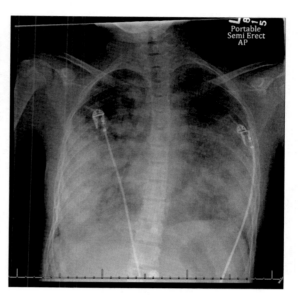

**Figure 2.** Chest radiograph showing multifocal airspace opacities.

requiring a transfusion of packed red blood cells. The rash continues to spread to her arms, prompting concern for a rickettsial infection, which prompted initiation of doxycycline. Her respiratory failure worsens, requiring transfer to the PICU on bilevel positive airway pressure and subsequent mechanical intubation. Repeated urine microscopy 4 days later demonstrates an increase of 21 to 50 red blood cells and new findings of proteinuria, with a urine protein/creatinine ratio of 1 (reference range, <0.2) in a spot and 24-hour collection. A chemistry panel showed a serum creatinine level of 0.51 mg/dL (45.08 μmol/L; reference range, 0.5–0.8 mg/dL [44.20–70.72 μmol/L]) and an estimated glomerular filtration rate of 145 mL/min per 1.73 m² (reference range, >90 mL/min per 1.73 m²). She acutely develops bloody oral secretions on day 5, and the respiratory support escalates to an oscillator. A concern for fungal involvement due to worsening hemoptysis despite broad antibiotic coverage expands her treatment to include amphotericin B. Her worsening respiratory failure and the anemia necessitate placement on extracorporeal membrane oxygenation. A bronchoscopy performed on day 6 demonstrates diffuse active bleeding.

## DISCUSSION

### Differential Diagnosis

The bilateral infiltrates in conjunction with the patient's hypoxemia and respiratory failure were initially concerning for an infectious process. However, the severe drop in hemoglobin concentration along with hemoptysis

suggested that the infiltrates seen on imaging were more consistent with diffuse alveolar hemorrhage (DAH). DAH develops when the damaged alveoli collect blood, disrupting gas exchange and resulting in acute respiratory failure. (1)

Infectious and autoimmune processes were the top 2 potential causes of lung injury in our patient. The infectious etiologies include *Streptococcus pneumonia, Staphylococcus aureus, Streptococcus pyogenes, Moraxella catarrhalis,* and *Haemophilus influenzae.* The addition of amphotericin B to our patient's regimen was due to concern for pulmonary

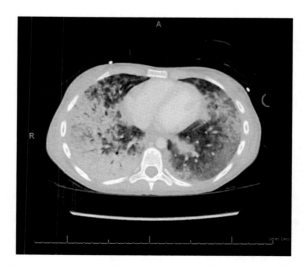

**Figure 3.** Chest computed tomographic scan showing air space consolidation with superimposed ground glass opacities.

histoplasmosis, which has been associated with DAH. (2) This patient presented before the COVID-19 pandemic, and, therefore, COVID-19 virus and subsequent multisystem inflammatory syndrome in children were not included in the differential diagnoses. The patient's low weight prompted an evaluation for an underlying primary immunodeficiency that revealed mild lymphopenia and low complement levels.

The possible etiologies of the erythematous macules included infectious and autoimmune processes. Suspicion for bacterial sepsis complicated by disseminated intravascular coagulation (DIC) was high because fulminant bacterial sepsis accounts for 95% of cases of DIC in children. (3) For the diagnosis of DIC, laboratory evaluation demonstrates an elevated D-dimer level, thrombocytopenia, a prolonged prothrombin time, and a decreased fibrinogen level. The resultant coagulopathy manifests as purpura, petechiae, or erythematous macules. (3) Our patient's elevated D-dimer level and prolonged prothrombin time suggested DIC. However, her elevated platelet count and fibrinogen level were not consistent with DIC, suggesting an alternate process. Other infectious causes of the rash that were considered included *Mycoplasma pneumoniae, Erlichia, Anaplasma, Coxiella burnetti, and Rickettsia typhi*. The prevalence of endemic typhus in Houston, Texas, made this entity highly suspect because it can present with skin findings described as nonpruritic, macular, or maculopapular rashes with a centrifugal spread originating from the trunk. (4) However, a typhus rash typically spares the palms and soles, unlike our patient's rash, which involved her palms. Initiation of empirical doxycycline in our patient addressed these etiologies while waiting for further results.

The autoimmune diseases that were considered based on her pulmonary-renal presentation and macular rash included antineutrophil cytoplasmic antibody (ANCA)–associated vasculitis, Goodpasture syndrome, systemic lupus erythematosus, antiphospholipid antibody syndrome, and mixed connective tissue disease. ANCA-associated vasculitides include granulomatosis with polyangiitis (GPA, formerly known as Wegener granulomatosis), microscopic polyangiitis, and eosinophilic granulomatosis with polyangiitis (formerly known as Churg-Strauss syndrome). The cutaneous manifestations of autoimmune rheumatic diseases are many, including macular erythematous rash, palpable purpura, tender subcutaneous nodules, oral and skin ulcerations, livedo reticularis, and Raynaud phenomenon, among others. (5) The serologic evaluation sent included an antinuclear antibody profile, anti–glomerular

basement membrane, an antiphospholipid antibody panel, and antiprothrombin antibodies, in addition to ANCA IgG, myeloperoxidase antibody, and serine proteinase 3 levels, which ultimately led to the diagnosis.

## Actual Diagnosis

Our patient exhibited an elevated serine proteinase 3 level of 954 U (reference range, <19 U) and an ANCA IgG titer of 1:2,560 (reference range, <1:20). A renal biopsy showed pauci-immune glomerulonephritis with 50% cellular crescents and mild interstitial fibrosis with predominantly interstitial edema. These findings confirmed the diagnosis of GPA.

## The Condition

GPA is an uncommon disorder that causes inflammation in the small blood vessels and involves the upper and lower respiratory tract as well as the kidneys. This systemic vasculitis is necrotizing and granulomatous, with local destruction of the involved organs. GPA results from an immune dysregulation and an environmental trigger in individuals with a genetic predisposition. (6) Other organ systems can be involved, including the central nervous system, the ocular system, and the skin. Pediatric GPA has a prevalence of 3.4 per 1,000,000 person-years and an incidence of 1.8 per 1,000,000 person-years. (7) It has a female predominance at a mean age of 14 years and a high probability of hospitalization at the time of diagnosis. Pediatric GPA usually presents with respiratory involvement and constitutional symptoms (fatigue, weight loss, and fever). (6) The diagnosis requires the fulfillment of at least 3 features from the European League Against Rheumatism/Paediatric Rheumatology International Trials Organisation/Paediatric Rheumatology European Society criteria (Table). (6)

Pediatric GPA often presents with upper airway or lower respiratory tract disease. The most common symptoms include shortness of breath, a chronic cough, and wheezing. (2) Hemoptysis as a manifestation of DAH occurs in 42% of patients with GPA. (2) One of the identified risk factors for development of DAH is hypocomplementemia. (8) A retrospective study of patients with ANCA-associated vasculitis demonstrated higher rates of DAH in patients with hypocomplementemia versus patients without hypocomplementemia (38% vs 8%; *P* = .007). (8) Interestingly, hemoptysis may be a late finding in one-third of patients with GPA. (1) The most common radiographic abnormalities in GPA are single or multiple nodular lesions, followed by fixed infiltrates and cavities. (9) In patients with a pulmonary hemorrhage, however, diffuse

**Table.** EULAR/PRINTO/PRES Criteria for Granulomatosis with Polyangiitis

**DIAGNOSTIC CRITERIA FOR PEDIATRIC GRANULOMATOSIS WITH POLYANGIITIS**

| | |
|---|---|
| ANCA positivity | Positive myeloperoxidase/p or serine proteinase 3/c-ANCA by immunofluorescence or by ELISA |
| Upper airway involvement | Chronic bloody or purulent nasal discharge or recurrent/chronic sinus inflammation |
| Pulmonary involvement | Radiologic evidence of nodules, cavities, or fixed infiltrates |
| Renal involvement | Proteinuria: >0.3 g/24 h or urine albumin/creatinine ratio >30 mmol/mg and/or |
| | Hematuria or RBC casts: >5 RBCs/HPF or RBCs in urine sediment or >2+ on dipstick or |
| | Necrotizing pauci-immune glomerulonephritis on renal histologic analysis |
| Histopathology | Arterial or arteriolar granulomatous inflammation in the artery wall or in perivascular or extravascular space on tissue biopsy (lung, skin, or kidney) |
| Laryngotracheobronchial stenosis | Subglottic, tracheal, or bronchial stenosis |

Three of the 6 criteria are required for diagnosis. (3) ANCA=antineutrophil cytoplasmic antibody, ELISA=enzyme-linked immunosorbent assay, EULAR/PRINTO/PRES=European League Against Rheumatism/Paediatric Rheumatology International Trials Organisation/Paediatric Rheumatology European Society, HPF=high-power field, RBC=red blood cell.

alveolar and interstitial opacities are the most common imaging findings. (2) For patients with an insidious presentation, evaluation with a pulmonary function test may be helpful. An obstructive pattern on a pulmonary function test is common, although 1 study found restrictive and obstructive patterns in equal proportion. (10) Often, a reduction in the diffusing lung capacity for carbon monoxide can be the first indication of a pulmonary hemorrhage, although this has not been validated. (2)

The renal involvement in GPA is a significant source of morbidity and mortality. The initial findings include urinary sediment abnormality, mild renal dysfunction, or acute kidney injury. (11) Fifty-seven percent of pediatric patients present with a significant acute kidney injury, defined as a glomerular filtration rate less than 60 mL/min per 1.73 m² and/or nephrotic-range proteinuria. (11) Our patient initially presented with hematuria with absent proteinuria and a normal serum creatinine level. Thus, the suspicion for glomerular involvement was initially low. However, the proteinuria on subsequent urine microscopies revealed the renal involvement. The gold standard for the diagnosis of ANCA-associated glomerulonephritis is a renal biopsy with findings of pauci-immune crescentic necrotizing glomerulonephritis. (11) Cellular crescents are associated with an improvement in renal function independent of the baseline glomerular filtration rate. (11) Poor renal outcomes are associated with fibrous crescents, glomerular sclerosis, and tubular atrophy, along with the degree of proteinuria. (11)

Treatment and Management

The treatment of GPA consists of an induction phase with high-dose corticosteroids with rituximab or pulse cyclophosphamide and a maintenance phase with rituximab or azathioprine or methotrexate with tapering doses of prednisone. (12) The induction phase is 3 to 6 months, and maintenance treatment can last 18 to 24 months. The induction treatment has significantly improved outcomes, but relapses are common, and many patients require repeated induction treatments, with medication-related toxicity. A combination of rituximab and cyclophosphamide as initial treatment can be considered for patients with a severe presentation, including life-threatening DAH and rapidly progressive glomerulonephritis. (2)

Without treatment, GPA has a 1-year mortality rate of up to 80% that is attributed to active vasculitis, renal insufficiency, and infection. (7) However, the adverse events related to the standard treatments also account for more than 50% of the 1-year mortality rate. (13) The long-term use of glucocorticoids is associated with increased infections, diabetes mellitus, gastrointestinal bleeding, and end-organ damage. (14) More recently, avacopan has been studied as a potential targeted therapy in lieu of glucocorticoids. (13) ANCA-associated vasculitis is thought to result from the complement component 5a binding to the complement component 5a receptor, resulting in inflammation. (13)(14) Avacopan selectively binds to the complement component 5a receptor, blocking complement activation. Two phase 2 studies suggest that avacopan is tolerated and comparable with glucocorticoids in clinical efficacy with an improved safety profile. (15) At the time of this submission, a larger phase 3 trial is in progress to investigate the long-term remission rates in the treatment of ANCA-associated vasculitis with avacopan. (13)

Patient Course

The patient received pulse methylprednisolone, 30 mg/kg intravenously (IV) 3 times, and plasmapheresis due to the pulmonary hemorrhage and continued extracorporeal membrane oxygenation for 6 days. She continued to have hemoptysis while intubated, so additional plasmapheresis was performed for a total of 7 sessions. After completing 7 days of plasmapheresis and IV immunoglobulin, 2 g/kg, she was given daily prednisone at an initial dose of 2 mg/kg per day and methylprednisolone, 30 mg/kg IV weekly, for 8 weeks; rituximab, 350 mg/m² per dose IV every week for 4 weeks; and cyclophosphamide, 500 mg/m² per dose monthly for 4 months. She completed a 14-day course of ceftriaxone and clindamycin for community-acquired pneumonia. Amphotericin B was discontinued after the fungal cultures were negative. She remained on trimethoprim-sulfamethoxazole for *Pneumocystis jirovecii* prophylaxis. She also received leuprolide for menstrual suppression during the cyclophosphamide treatment to preserve ovarian function and future fertility. (16)(17) She transitioned to a maintenance regimen with azathioprine and low-dose prednisone. She has since been able to restart school with close follow-up with the rheumatology, renal, and pulmonary services. She remains in clinical remission 15 months after initial presentation.

## Lessons for the Clinician

- Although rare in children, antineutrophil cytoplasmic antibody–associated vasculitis should be considered in patients presenting with hypoxemia and imaging suggestive of pneumonia that does not improve with empirical antibiotics.
- Diffuse alveolar hemorrhage can mimic pneumonia on imaging and should be considered in the setting of acutely worsening anemia and respiratory distress.
- Renal involvement is common in systemic vasculitis and prone to relapses despite early aggressive therapy.
- A multidisciplinary approach should be used when initial diagnostic assessments do not progress as expected.

*References for this article can be found at*
https://doi.org/10.1542/pir.2021-005011.

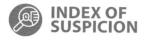

INDEX OF
SUSPICION

# Respiratory Distress and Weight Loss in a 16-year-old Boy with a History of Pancreatitis

Alexander Bowers, DO,* Nicholas Friedman, DO,* Jason Caboot, MD*

*Department of Pediatrics, Madigan Army Medical Center, Tacoma, WA

## PRESENTATION

A 16-year-old Asian American male with a history of recurrent pancreatitis (4 episodes since 4 years of age) and sinusitis (last episode around age 6 years) presents to his primary care physician with a persistent, productive cough, fatigue, and dyspnea for 2 months after being hospitalized and treated for community-acquired and eventually atypical pneumonia with ampicillin and azithromycin 1 month previously. In addition, he endorses a 15-lb weight loss over that time. His examination is significant for increased work of breathing with nasal flaring. Rhonchi are auscultated in bilateral bases of his lungs. No significant sinus tenderness, palpable lymphadenopathy, additional heart sounds or murmurs, abdominal tenderness, or edema was appreciated. His electrolyte and liver enzyme levels are normal. His white blood cell count is 14,000/μL ($14 \times 10^9$/L), with a normal differential cell count. Chest radiographs (Figs 1 and 2) show increased bilateral perihilar markings with a right middle lobe infiltrate and an obscured cardiac silhouette. A chest computed tomographic scan (Fig 3) is obtained and shows diffuse bronchiectasis. Pulmonology is consulted for bronchoscopy with bronchoalveolar lavage (BAL), which reveals edematous bronchial mucosa and thick, purulent secretions. Respiratory cultures from the BAL fluid grow *Staphylococcus aureus* and *Aspergillus fumigatus*. Total serum immunoglobulin E (IgE) and serum *A fumigatus* IgE levels are both elevated (>19,000 IU/mL and 50,000 kU/L, respectively). An interferon-based tuberculosis test is obtained and the results are negative. Blood cultures are negative after 5 days.

With his history of recurrent pancreatitis and sinusitis, he was previously evaluated for cystic fibrosis (CF) via sweat chloride testing at 7 years old, with borderline results of 40 mEq/L (40 mmol/L). A full familial pancreatitis panel and cystic fibrosis transmembrane conductor regulator (CFTR) genetic testing were also performed at follow-up with his gastrointestinal physician when the patient was 14 years old and was having continued abdominal pain with episodes of pancreatitis. He was found to have a heterozygote single *CFTR* mutation, c.3717+1G>T, of unknown significance.

He is hospitalized and started on broad spectrum antibiotics with concern for bilateral pneumonia.

## DIAGNOSIS

With the growth of aspergillus on sputum cultures and the elevated levels of both total IgE and aspergillus antibody IgE, a diagnosis of acute bronchopulmonary

**AUTHOR DISCLOSURE** Drs Bowers, Friedman, and Caboot have disclosed no financial relationships relevant to this article. This commentary does not contain a discussion of an unapproved/investigative use of a commercial product/device. The views expressed are those of the authors and do not reflect the official policy of the Department of the Army, the Department of Defense, or the US Government.

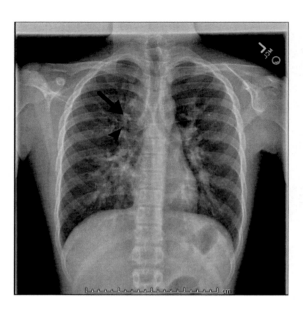

**Figure 1.** The patient's posteroanterior chest radiograph demonstrating suprahilar densities (arrow) consistent with bronchiectasis and mucous plugging (arrowhead).

aspergillosis (ABPA) was made. Given the diffuse bronchiectasis and diagnosis of ABPA, there was concern again for CF. The prevalence of aspergillus colonization in CF has been reported to be as high as 65% of cases. (1) Repeated sweat chloride testing was performed (borderline elevated values of 47 and 52 mEq/L [47 and 52 mmol/L]). Based on sweat chloride levels and genetic analysis, the patient did not

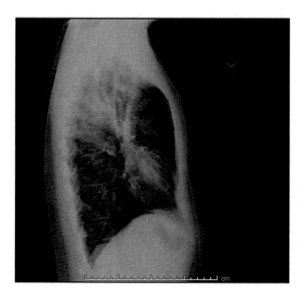

**Figure 2.** The patient's lateral chest radiograph demonstrating suprahilar densities consistent with bronchiectasis and mucous plugging (arrowhead).

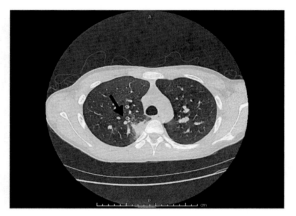

**Figure 3.** The patient's chest computed tomographic scan demonstrating bronchiectasis, bronchial wall thickening, and mucous plugging (arrow).

meet the diagnostic criteria for CF. The patient was diagnosed as having a CFTR-related disorder based on the genotypic evaluation and phenotypic presentation. Testicular ultrasonography revealed the presence of bilateral vas deferens.

## The Condition

CF is the most common multisystem autosomal recessive disorder in the United States, affecting 1:3,000 white people and 1:30,000 Asian American people. When clinical suspicion for CF is high but sweat chloride results are inconclusive, DNA sequencing can assess for *CFTR* mutations. The gene for the CFTR is located on chromosome 7 and encodes an ion channel protein. If a patient has pathology consistent with CF, does not meet the strict diagnostic criteria (elevation of sweat chloride level, 2 *CFTR* mutations), but does have at least 1 mutation in the *CFTR* gene, a CFTR-related disorder may be diagnosed. (2) There are a variety of disease processes that are known to be affected by the CFTR genotype but that do not meet the diagnostic criteria for CF. The most prominent of these are congenital bilateral absence of the vas deferens, acute recurrent or chronic pancreatitis, chronic rhinosinusitis, and diffuse bronchiectasis. Typically, only 1 organ system is involved in such patients. Approximately 30% of patients with idiopathic chronic pancreatitis or acute recurrent pancreatitis have a *CFTR* mutation, and 10% to 50% of patients with bronchiectasis have at least 1 *CFTR* mutation. (3)(4) No single mutation is exclusively associated with this disorder, but cases often cite mutations of the IVF8-5T allele on the *CFTR* gene as opposed to the F508del mutation most commonly cited in CF. (3)(5) In addition, CF is a relatively uncommon diagnosis in patients of Asian ancestry. The most prevalent Asian countries with cases of CF include those in the Middle East to include Jordan and Bahrain. Countries such as Japan have a CF incidence of 1:350,000, and China has reported only 30 cases as of 2015. (6) The prevalence of CFTR-related disorders in patients with Asian ancestry is unknown. Our patient's mother is Filipino and his father is Vietnamese and Chinese. A comparative analysis of the CFTR2 database did determine that Asian patients with CF, compared with those of Eastern European ancestry, often have a higher percentage of sweat chloride results less than 60 mEq/L (<60 mmol/L) (14% versus 6%), a lower percentage of homozygous F508del mutations (17.2 versus 46.1%), and a higher percentage of pancreatic-sufficient disease (24.9 versus 17.1%). (7)

## Management

As with CF, CFTR-related disorders incorporate a wide spectrum of different pathologies with varying degrees of dysfunction. Therefore, no single-target management routine is possible. With CFTR-related disorders, typically only 1 organ system is affected, so management can often be more focused. As in our case, if the primary pathology is pulmonary in nature, an appropriate pulmonary clearance regimen is needed to decrease the risk of exacerbations. In those with recurrent or chronic pancreatitis as their phenotypic presentation, supportive therapy for pancreatitis is often needed. As opposed to CF, relatively few patients have exocrine pancreatic insufficiency and, therefore, do not require supplemental pancreatic enzyme therapy. (3) Unfortunately, this patient population does not currently qualify for treatment with the CFTR modulating therapies.

## Patient Course

The patient was admitted to the hospital and started on intravenous antibiotics, initially broad coverage with gentamicin and ceftazidime and eventually narrowed to nafcillin after BAL revealed pan-sensitive methicillin-sensitive *Staphylococcus aureus*. For the treatment of his ABPA, he was started on oral itraconazole and prednisone. Throughout his 2-week hospitalization, he performed frequent airway clearance therapy with albuterol, hypertonic saline, and vest therapy in a similar way that a CF exacerbation would be managed. His energy and cough greatly improved, and he began to have weight gain. Serial pulmonary function tests were performed and demonstrated severe obstructive pulmonary disease, consistent with ABPA, and had bronchodilator response that improved throughout his admission. He was discharged on a prolonged course of itraconazole and prednisone that was weaned by pediatric pulmonology as his IgE levels improved over the course of several months. He continued on home airway clearance after discharge. He has had no further recurrences of ABPA, pneumonia, or other pulmonary exacerbations of his CFTR-related disorder but has had additional episodes of pancreatitis.

## Lessons for the Clinician

- Although there are strict diagnostic criteria for cystic fibrosis, much less is known about the broad genotypic and phenotypic spectrum of cystic fibrosis transmembrane conductor regulator (CFTR)–related disorders.
- Diagnosis is determined by characteristic phenotypic pathology, indeterminate sweat chloride test results, and the presence of at least 1 mutation in the *CFTR* gene.
- Multisystem disease is uncommon in a patient with a CFTR-related disorder.
- Cystic fibrosis is a relatively uncommon diagnosis in patients of Asian ancestry, and the prevalence of CFTR-related disorders is unknown.

*References for this article can be found at*
https://doi.org/10.1542/pir.2020-0084

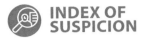

INDEX OF
SUSPICION

# Respiratory Distress in a Newborn: Who Nose?

CPT Kyle Sunshein, MD,* CPT Matthew Nestander, MD,† Maj Stephanie Eighmy, DO†

*Department of Pediatrics, Brooke Army Medical Center, Fort Sam Houston, TX
†Department of Pediatrics, Neonatal Division, Brooke Army Medical Center, Fort Sam Houston, TX

## PRESENTATION

A term female infant develops new onset respiratory distress at 6 hours of age in the newborn nursery. She was born via spontaneous vaginal delivery and only required routine stimulation during initial resuscitation. Apgar scores were 8 and 9 at 1 and 5 minutes of age, respectively. Her prenatal course was uncomplicated, and maternal serologies were negative for infectious risk factors. The initial physical examination after birth revealed a well-appearing, non-dysmorphic neonate in no apparent distress. On repeat examination at 6 hours of age, the infant exhibits tachypnea, intercostal retractions, nasal flaring, and an unusual, high-pitched inspiratory stertor with whistling. On close auscultation, this sound is appreciated best over the left nostril. Her lungs are clear to auscultation bilaterally. No external facial or nasal malformations are noted. No appreciable heart murmurs are heard on cardiac examination. Pulse oximetry shows intermittent desaturation as low as 85% on room air with concordant upper and lower extremity measurements. The infant is transferred to intensive care for further evaluation and respiratory support.

Continuous cardiorespiratory monitoring reveals continued intermittent desaturations that are most notable at rest. Of note, the desaturations improve quickly when the infant cries. A chest radiograph reveals clear lung fields bilaterally and a normal cardiac silhouette. The infant continues to exhibit loud nasal stertor and whistling throughout her initial evaluation. A 5 French nasogastric tube is passed successfully through the right nostril, but the tube is unable to pass through the left nostril because of notable resistance. This finding raises suspicion for an upper airway obstruction, and pediatric otolaryngology is consulted to assist in the evaluation. Flexible endoscopy of the infant's nasal passages and subsequent computed tomography of the sinuses eventually confirm the final diagnosis.

## DISCUSSION

### Differential Diagnosis

The vast majority of cases of neonatal respiratory distress are because of pathology involving the lower respiratory tract. The etiologies involving the upper respiratory tract, specifically the nasal passages, are not as extensive and were the main focus of our evaluation given the infant's unusual respiratory sounds and questionable nasal patency. Because neonates are considered to be obligate nasal breathers at rest, crying with an open mouth allows them to bypass potential nasal obstruction to improve gas exchange. The normalization of oxygen saturation during episodes of crying in our patient provided a valuable clinical clue.

AUTHOR DISCLOSURE: Drs Sunshein, Nestander, and Eighmy disclose no financial conflicts of interest. The views expressed herein are those of the authors and do not reflect the official policy or position of Brooke Army Medical Center, the US Army Medical Department, the US Army Office of the Surgeon General, the Department of the Army, the Department of the Air Force, or the Department of Defense or the US government.

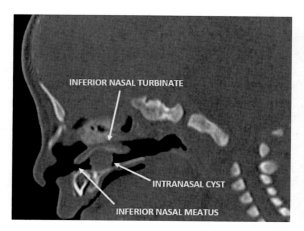

**Figure 1.** Sagittal computed tomography view of an intranasal cyst arising from a congenital dacryocystocele. The distal portion of the cyst is shown extending into and obstructing the left nasal passage.

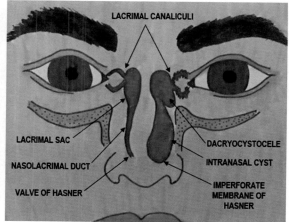

**Figure 2.** Anatomic illustration of the normal nasolacrimal apparatus (left) and a congenital dacryocystocele (right). The persistent membrane of Hasner results in fluid accumulation and cystic expansion of the lacrimal sac. This leads to a functional compression of the lacrimal canaliculi and a resulting closed cyst space. Distal mucosal expansion forms an intranasal cyst that can obstruct the nasal passage. Proximal and distal cystic swelling connected by a narrower nasolacrimal duct creates a dumbbell-shaped mass that can be seen on imaging. (Reprinted with permission from Sunshein S. [2021]. Dacryocystocele Anatomic Diagram).

Choanal atresia is a rare but well-recognized anatomic defect involving membranous or bony blockage of the posterior nasal passages. Bilateral choanal atresia leads to notable upper airway obstruction and respiratory distress in newborns, whereas unilateral choanal atresia is milder and may present later in life. Masses such as hemangiomas, lymphangiomas, mucoceles, dermoid cysts, dacryocystoceles, and encephaloceles are also potential causes of unilateral nasal obstruction.

## Actual Diagnosis

Flexible endoscopy performed by pediatric otolaryngology reveals a pale-colored nasal mass just under the left inferior turbinate. Computed tomography of the sinuses shows a dumbbell-shaped soft tissue mass within the left nasolacrimal duct suggestive of a congenital dacryocystocele with cystic extension into the nasal passage (Fig 1).

## The Condition

Physiologic nasolacrimal drainage is facilitated by the canalization of an embryological structure called the membrane of Hasner at the distal nasolacrimal duct. This process typically occurs before or shortly after birth to form the valve of Hasner. Congenital dacryocystocele, a rare variant of congenital nasolacrimal duct obstruction, occurs when this membrane persists and leads to a distal anatomic obstruction of nasolacrimal drainage. A resulting backflow of fluid leads to cystic expansion of the lacrimal sac and adjacent mucosa. Proximal compression of the lacrimal canaliculi by this cyst is theorized to create a one-way valve effect leading to further collection of mucoid fluid that can extend distally into the nasal passage (Fig 2). (1)(2)

The incidence of congenital dacryocystocele is estimated to be one in three thousand eight hundred and eighty-four live births or ~0.02%. It is usually unilateral and presents more commonly in female infants. (3) The diagnosis is classically suggested by a bluish skin swelling near the medial canthus, but this is not always present on physical examination. In fact, infants without this classic examination finding are usually diagnosed after an associated complication arises. (3)(4) The gold-standard imaging technique for this diagnosis is computed tomography of the sinuses. Endoscopy and ultrasonography are alternative options that do not involve radiation but are less sensitive. (5) Although many infants with dacryocystoceles do not develop symptoms, notable complications can arise from this anatomic variant. Stasis of cyst contents can lead to infections in the form of dacryocystitis and cellulitis. Respiratory distress is a less commonly observed complication affecting 9.5% to 17% of infants with dacryocystoceles. (2)(4) Because infants are known to be obligate nasal breathers, enlarged dacryocystoceles that extend into the nasal passages can create an obstruction notable enough to produce respiratory distress. (6)

## Treatment and Management

Once the diagnosis is suspected, management largely depends on the individual symptoms and degree of nasal obstruction. Establishing appropriate respiratory support should be the immediate priority in cases involving respiratory symptoms. Consultation with otolaryngology can be considered in cases that require airway intervention. Urgent ophthalmology referral is warranted to determine the need for surgical intervention. In stable or asymptomatic patients, outpatient observation is reasonable to assess for spontaneous resolution, which occurs in 23% to 33% of cases, usually within the first month of age. This is theorized to occur because of spontaneous perforation of the membrane of Hasner to form a patent nasolacrimal duct. (2)(3) Crigler massage, the act of exerting downward digital pressure on the external portion of the lacrimal sac, may be effective at relieving the obstruction. (4) Parents should be instructed on proper massage technique to help promote lacrimal drainage while being followed periodically by ophthalmology. Intranasal steroids were used to alleviate local swelling of the nasal turbinates after endoscopy in our case, but there are no data supporting their long-term use for this condition. The risk of dacryocystitis and cellulitis is high in persistent dacryocystoceles, and treatment of these complications warrants intravenous antibiotics and potential surgical intervention. These infectious complications typically present within the first 2 to 3 months of age. (2)(3)(7) Preferred surgical options for this lesion include endoscopic-assisted nasolacrimal probing or cyst marsupialization. Both procedures involve perforation of the intranasal cyst to achieve nasolacrimal duct patency and allow proper drainage. (1)(7)

### Patient Course

Because of her intermittent hypoxemia on admission, low flow oxygen was briefly used via facemask. Humidified high-flow nasal cannula was considered because of her initial increased work of breathing; however, this was not required because of gradual improvement in respiratory effort. A nasal trumpet and intubation supplies were kept at the bedside in case of worsening respiratory distress. Pediatric ophthalmology was consulted as soon as the diagnosis was made for further assistance in management. Treatment was initiated with intranasal dexamethasone drops to alleviate associated swelling. Surgical marsupialization of the cyst was strongly considered given her respiratory symptoms after birth. However, her clinical status gradually improved over the first 48 hours of age with conservative management alone. She was able to tolerate breastfeeding well, without notable desaturations or respiratory distress. No further vital sign abnormalities were observed during the remainder of her hospitalization. She was discharged from the hospital in stable condition and was followed closely as an outpatient by her general clinician and ophthalmologist. No infectious complications were noted over the span of 2 months, after which, follow-up information was unavailable.

### Lessons for the Clinician

- Improvement in respiratory status of a neonate during episodes of crying, with relative worsening at rest, could suggest a nasal obstruction.
- Congenital dacryocystocele is an uncommon anatomic defect of the nasolacrimal duct. Although they are commonly asymptomatic and self-resolving, they can present with nasal obstruction and respiratory distress in newborns.
- Common infectious complications of dacryocystoceles include dacryocystitis and cellulitis, both of which require intravenous antibiotics and possible surgical intervention.
- The diagnosis is suggested by the classic finding of a bluish skin swelling near the medial canthus. Endoscopy or radiologic imaging can be used to confirm the diagnosis.
- It is important for pediatric clinicians to recognize this condition as well as the associated complications to promptly involve a pediatric ophthalmologist in management.

*References for this article can be found at*
https://doi.org/10.1542/pir.2021-005313

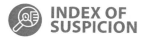

# Seven-Year-Old Girl with Fever and Abdominal Pain

Cindy D. Chang, MD,*† Payton Thode, MD,‡ Lindsey Barrick, DO, MPH*§

*Division of Emergency Medicine, Cincinnati Children's Hospital Medical Center, Cincinnati, OH
†Department of Emergency Medicine, University of Cincinnati Medical Center, Cincinnati, OH
‡Department of Emergency Medicine, Morton Hospital, Taunton, MA
§Department of Pediatrics, University of Cincinnati School of Medicine, Cincinnati, OH

## PRESENTATION

A healthy, fully immunized, 7-year-old girl presents to the emergency department (ED) with right-sided abdominal pain since the morning of presentation. She vomited once and was febrile to 101°F (38.3°C) at school. Her brother was sick the previous week with fever, headache, and vomiting that resolved. An ultrasonography reveals a normal appendix, her flu test result is negative, and she is discharged from the hospital with presumed viral gastroenteritis. The fevers continue, and 3 days later, the patient represents to the ED for respiratory distress.

The patient's mother reports that, throughout the previous night, the patient developed new and worsening difficulty breathing. She woke up frequently, complaining of chest and right upper abdominal pain. There were no rashes, joint swelling, recent traveling, or ingestion.

At ED arrival, physical examination reveals an awake, alert, ill-appearing patient sitting upright in bed in moderate respiratory distress. Her vital signs are temperature, 102.2°F (39°C); heart rate, 168 beats/min; respiration rate, 60 breaths/min; blood pressure, 94/79 mm Hg; and pulse oxygen saturation ($S_{PO_2}$), 97% on room air. The patient's head, neck, eyes, ears, nose, and throat reveal an erythematous throat with no tonsillar exudates, dry mucous membranes, and shotty anterior cervical adenopathy. She is tachycardic without murmurs and with a capillary refill of 4 seconds. She is tachypneic with diminished breath sounds in the right lower base. Her abdomen is soft but tender to palpation in the right upper quadrant without peritoneal signs or hepatosplenomegaly; she has no costovertebral angle tenderness. She has a diffuse, blanching, fine, erythematous papular, scarlatiniform rash over the upper extremities and torso. The rash was not sunburn-like in appearance, and no peeling was noted. Her mental status is normal. Ten minutes after examination, her $S_{PO_2}$ drops to 89%, and she is placed on 2 L of $O_2$ via nasal cannula with improvement to 96%.

Diagnostics in the ED reveal the following values (reference ranges): venous blood gas while on 2 L nasal cannula with pH, 7.43 (7.35–7.45); $Pa_{CO_2}$, 32 mm Hg (45–55 mm Hg); bicarbonate, 21.4 mmol/L (22–28 mmol/L); and base excess, −3 mmol/L (+/−2 mmol/L). A basic metabolic panel reveals the following abnormal values (reference ranges): sodium, 129 mmol/L (136–145 mmol/L); and chloride, 98 mmol/L (100–112 mmol/L). Potassium, bicarbonate, anion gap, blood urea nitrogen, creatinine, and glucose were normal. A complete blood cell count reveals the following abnormal values (reference ranges): white blood cell (WBC) count 26.95 (5.00–14.5 × 10³/mcL) with a differential that is remarkable; elevated segmented neutrophils of 85.2% (40.0%–46.0%); and normal band cells at 2.6% (0.0%–4.0%). Hemoglobin,

AUTHOR DISCLOSURE: Drs Chang, Thode, and Barrick have no financial relationships that could be broadly relevant to the work.

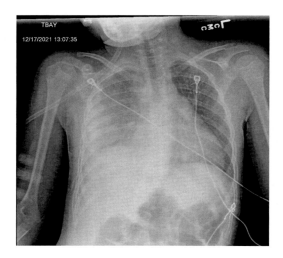

**Figure 1.** Anteroposterior chest radiograph revealing opacification of the right hemithorax.

hematocrit, mean corpuscular volume, and platelet count are normal. Other inflammatory markers are notable for the following (reference ranges): erythrocyte sedimentation rate, 31 mm/h (0–10 mm/h); C-reactive protein, 30.3 mg/dL (normal range ≤0.40 mg/dL); lactic acid level, 2.45 mmol/L (0.90–2.10 mmol/L); procalcitonin, 46.70 ng/mL (<0.5 ng/mL indicates that systemic infection is not likely); and lactate dehydrogenase, 303 U/L (135–395 U/L). Influenza A and B and SARS-CoV-2 test results are negative. Liver function tests, lipase, and urinalysis are normal. A rapid antigen-based group A *Streptococcus* (GAS) swab from her throat yields a positive result.

A portable anteroposterior chest radiograph (Fig 1) reveals "opacification of right hemithorax, in part owing to a moderate size right pleural effusion. Underlying airspace disease is suspected. Pneumonia is possible." Ultrasonography of the chest reveals "moderate/large simple right pleural effusion with associated atelectasis of the right lung."

The patient is given a 20 mL/kg intravenous (IV) fluid bolus and started on ampicillin. She improves in the ED and is admitted to the floor.

## DISCUSSION

### Differential Diagnosis

On her first presentation, with the complaints of abdominal pain and fever, clinicians focused on infectious abdominal pathology, specifically appendicitis. Other infectious etiologies of abdominal pain include mesenteric adenitis, urinary tract infections, gastroenteritis, and occult pneumonia. As her disease progressed, the differential diagnosis expanded. Physical examination findings of respiratory distress, unilateral

diminished breath sounds, and hypoxia localize to a lung cause as the source. The differential for a unilateral opacification on chest radiograph includes effusion, atelectasis or lung collapse, mainstem bronchial obstruction, tumor, and infectious consolidation.

Pleural effusions can lead to respiratory distress and be exudative or transudative. Transudative effusions are seen with heart failure, liver disease, and nephrotic syndrome. These are less likely without other clinical features of third spacing on examination. The concurrence of fevers and elevated inflammatory markers increased suspicion for infectious or malignant etiologies, with infectious being the most likely; exudative effusion was presumed. Most often associated with bacterial pneumonias, parapneumonic effusions can also be caused by viral, fungal, and atypical bacteria.

The patient had the clinical rash of scarlet fever, which prompted GAS antigen testing from the throat. The swab result was positive. She never complained of sore throat during this illness, and it is known that up to 20% of asymptomatic school-age children may be GAS carriers. [1][2] Distinguishing carrier status from active disease can be challenging, but it is important. Carriers rarely have complications of streptococcal disease, but active streptococcal pharyngitis can lead to nonsuppurative and suppurative complications if untreated. Nonsuppurative complications include toxic shock syndrome, acute glomerulonephritis, acute rheumatic fever, and poststreptococcal reactive arthritis. Suppurative complications include abscesses (tonsillar, brain), otitis medium, sinusitis, streptococcal bacteremia, necrotizing fasciitis, meningitis, and Lemierre syndrome.

### Actual Diagnosis

The patient initially responds to IV fluid resuscitation, supplemental oxygen, and fever reduction. Having clinically improved, she is admitted to the hospital floor with presumed community-acquired pneumonia complicated by a parapneumonic effusion. Within 2 hours, she develops worsening respiratory distress and hypoxia. Grunting and nasal flaring develop. Her respiratory rate increases from 32 to 52 breaths/min, and she requires 8 L of oxygen by mask to keep saturations greater than 90%. A chest/abdomen/pelvis computed tomography scan with contrast is performed and reveals the following: 1) a large loculated right pleural effusion with complete collapse of the right lower lobe, with obstruction of the right lower lobar bronchus, possibly because of extrinsic compression related to pleural effusion; and 2) patchy ground glass opacities in the right upper lobe, which could relate to edema, atelectasis, or pneumonia (Figs 2A and 2B). Antibiotics are broadened to include vancomycin and ceftriaxone. The patient is transferred to the

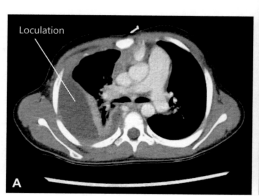

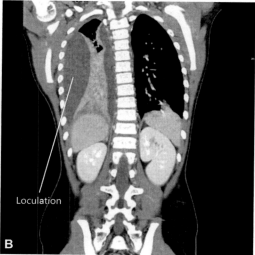

**Figure 2.** A. and B.: Computed tomography scan of chest and abdomen reveals a large loculated right pleural effusion with complete collapse of the right lower lobe.

PICU. A chest tube is placed, draining 20 mL of pleural fluid. Pleural fluid diagnostic studies reveal a turbid appearance; red blood cell count of 6,111 mm³; WBC count of 20,450 mm³; segmented neutrophils of 86%; band cells of 2%; lymphocytes of 3%; monocytes of 1%; eosinophils of 8%; protein of 4.6 gm/dL; and lactate dehydrogenase of 8,796 U/L. Gram-stain reveals many WBCs and few gram-positive cocci in pairs. Pleural fluid cultures grow few GAS, verifying the diagnosis of *Streptococcus* empyema.

The rapid development and progression of severe respiratory symptoms within 24 hours before her decompensation are consistent with a diagnosis of explosive pleuritis. Because the patient initially presented with neither a sore throat nor a cough, the inciting source of the GAS is unclear. With the concurrence of scarlet fever, a positive GAS antigen swab result from the pharynx, and a complicated pneumonia, the authors hypothesize that explosive pleuritis is an uncommon complication of GAS pharyngitis. The presenting tachycardia and poor perfusion suggest the early development of toxic shock syndrome, aborted by ampicillin.

## The Condition
Explosive pleuritis is a rare complication of GAS infection. It was described in a 1986 case report as a rapid development of pleural effusions involving more than 90% of the hemithorax. (3) The pathogenesis involves streptococcal cellular debris blocking peri-bronchial and subpleural lymphatics, which can cause compression of pulmonary tissue and mediastinal shift to the contralateral side. (4) GAS, also known as *Streptococcus pyogenes*, is a gram-positive coccus organism in chains.

Explosive pleuritis is essentially a rapidly progressive pleural empyema, and clinical features include hypoxia, respiratory distress, unilateral diminished breath sounds, and fever. Additional symptoms in adults include severe pharyngitis, persistent high fevers, intense pleuritic pain, and worsening respiratory distress. (3)(4)

The most common pathogen causing bacterial pneumonia and associated effusions is *Streptococcus pneumoniae*. Rates of *S pneumoniae* have been declining since the introduction of the seven-valent pneumococcal conjugate vaccine in 2000. (5)(6)(7) *Staphylococcus aureus* and other species of *Streptococcus* are also important causes of pneumonias associated with exudative effusions. Pleural fluid, when cultured, will grow the causative agent and contribute to the diagnosis.

Although they account for a small percentage of parapneumonic effusions, the association of effusions with pneumonia is much higher for GAS than other agents (10% other versus 80% GAS). (8)(9) Parapneumonic effusions associated with GAS disease are notable because of the rapid progression of the effusion, higher risks of complications, circulatory failure, respiratory disorders, chest tube drainage, and ICU admission. (3)(6)(10) Sixty-two percent of patients with a GAS pleural empyema present with a rash. (11) The incidence of invasive GAS disease, including parapneumonic effusions, is increasing globally and in the United States. (12)(13)(14)(15)(16)

## Treatment and Management
Patients with pleural fluid in the setting of a scarlatiniform rash require pleural fluid collection for cell count and culture and immediate antibiotics with penicillin agents. Consider

adding clindamycin for toxin control if streptococcal toxic shock syndrome is suspected. Early thoracentesis or chest tube placement is necessary for diagnostic and therapeutic purposes. If the patient does not improve or the effusion is loculated and does not adequately drain with a chest tube, consider drainage through thoracotomy or video-assisted thoracoscopic surgery for decortication and active drainage.

### Patient Course

During admission to the PICU, the patient developed worsening respiratory distress and required 8 L of $O_2$ to maintain saturations greater than 92%. After the chest tube was placed and the fluid drained, her respiratory status improved. She was continued on ceftriaxone monotherapy until the chest tube was removed on day 10 and then transitioned to amoxicillin. The patient was discharged from the hospital on day 13 on amoxicillin to complete a 21-day course.

### Lessons for the Clinician

- It is important to keep a broad differential when children present with fevers and abdominal pain.
- Clinical parapneumonic effusion with a scarlatiniform rash at presentation should increase concern for GAS and invasive disease, with high risk of circulatory compromise.
- Explosive pleuritis is a rare complication of GAS infection associated with rapid deterioration that requires antibiotics and prompt drainage.

*References for this article can be found at*
https://doi.org/10.1542/pir.2022-005912

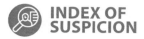

# INDEX OF SUSPICION

# Stridor in a 7-month-old Girl

Aoife Corcoran, MBBS,* Pelton Phinizy, MD,* Joe Piccione, DO, MS*

*Division of Pulmonary & Sleep Medicine, Children's Hospital of Philadelphia, University of Pennsylvania School of Medicine, Philadelphia, PA

## PRESENTATION

A 7-month-old former term, fully immunized girl with normal newborn screen results presents to the clinic with complaints of "noisy breathing" and cough.

Her "noisy breathing" has been present since birth and is worse with feeding and upper respiratory tract infections (URIs). She has no history of respiratory distress or intubation at birth. Her breathing became notably louder at 4 months of age. Her breathing is quiet during sleep, and her parents note snoring only when she has a URI. She also has a chronic cough that is worse in the morning and after feeding but also occurs in the absence of feeding. The quality of the cough is described as "barky or harsh." She has had three episodes of bronchiolitis during which the cough and "noisy breathing" worsened notably. She has been trialed on nebulized budesonide twice daily after her most recent bronchiolitis, which required hospital admission, with no improvement noted. There is a history of asthma and seasonal allergies in both of her parents.

She is feeding by mouth and is currently at the 50th percentile for weight, length, and weight-for-length. She is currently being treated empirically for gastroesophageal reflux disease with famotidine. She has no diarrhea or emesis and no cyanosis or sweating with feeding. She is non-dysmorphic and has been meeting all developmental milestones appropriately. On examination, she is noted to have harsh biphasic (inspiratory and expiratory) stridor but is breathing comfortably, with no retractions. Her cry is strong, with no hoarseness noted. Her vital signs show a heart rate of 123 beats/min, pulse oxygen saturation ($Spo_2$) of 97%, respiratory rate of 31 breaths/min, and blood pressure of 90/60 mmHg in clinic. An earlier chest radiograph obtained during one episode of bronchiolitis revealed mild peri-bronchial cuffing with no consolidation. A video fluoroscopic swallow study revealed trace laryngeal penetration with thin consistency barium without tracheal aspiration. She was electively scheduled for an airway evaluation involving microlaryngoscopy and rigid bronchoscopy by the otolaryngologists (ENTs), flexible bronchoscopy by pulmonologists, and esophagogastroduodenoscopy by the gastroenterologists (GIs), which revealed the diagnosis.

## DISCUSSION

### Differential Diagnosis

Stridor is caused by obstruction of the airway at the level of the larynx or trachea (Table 1). The timing of the stridor (inspiratory, expiratory, or biphasic) can be informative in assessing the level of airway obstruction. Inspiratory stridor occurs with an extra-thoracic obstruction at the glottic or supra-glottic level. Expiratory stridor occurs when there is an intrathoracic obstruction or compression. Biphasic

AUTHOR DISCLOSURES: Aoife Corcoran, MBBS, Pelton Phinizy, MD, and Joe Piccione, DO, MS, have disclosed no financial relationships relevant to this article. This commentary does not contain a discussion of an unapproved/investigative use of a commercial product/device.

**Table 1.** Common Causes of Chronic Stridor in Infants

| Location | Etiology |
|---|---|
| Larynx | Laryngomalacia |
| | Laryngeal web |
| | Laryngeal cyst |
| | Laryngeal cleft |
| | Subglottic hemangioma |
| | Subglottic stenosis |
| | Vocal cord papilloma |
| | Vocal cord paralysis |
| Trachea | Tracheal stenosis |
| | Complete tracheal rings |
| | Vascular rings and slings |
| | Tracheomalacia |

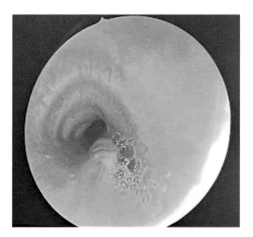

**Figure 1.** A 2- to 3-cm longitudinal ridge of tissue in the distal third of the trachea.

stridor is often indicative of notable, fixed airway obstruction at the level of the glottis, sub-glottis, or trachea. There have been rare cases in which variable obstruction in the supraglottis also causes biphasic stridor. History and physical exam findings play an important role in the evaluation of stridor. Laryngomalacia is by far the most common cause of stridor in infancy, at an estimated incidence of one in two thousand one hundred infants. (1) It is usually worse when the infant is supine and typically resolves without intervention by the second year postnatal (12–24 months of age). The quality of the infant's cry can be informative, suggesting the possibility of vocal cord injury, hypomobility, or a laryngeal web. In severe cases, gastroesophageal reflux disease can cause laryngeal and tracheal mucosal edema resulting in stridor. A history of intubation at birth would raise suspicions for acquired glottic or subglottic stenosis, and a history of recurrent URIs along with coughing with feeding would be concerning for a tracheoesophageal fistula (TEF) or posterior laryngeal cleft resulting in recurrent aspiration. Extrinsic compression of the airway (vascular rings) and masses within the airway (ie, hemangioma, foreign body) can cause stridor and/or wheezing. Complete tracheal rings are a rare, life-threatening anomaly that present with worsening stridor and respiratory distress as the patient grows. Complete tracheal rings are frequently associated with vascular rings.

Actual Diagnosis

The patient was taken for microlaryngoscopy and rigid bronchoscopy by the ENTs and flexible bronchoscopy by the pulmonologists, which revealed a 2- to 3-cm longitudinal ridge of tissue in the distal third of the trachea (Fig 1). The area was insufflated and examined extensively, with no signs of TEF. Mild tracheomalacia was noted in the distal trachea during the dynamic airway evaluation. Upper airway anatomy and lower tracheobronchial tree anatomy were both normal, with no evidence of stenosis or malacia. Esophagogastro-

duodenoscopy conducted by the GIs revealed a small area of extrinsic compression in the proximal esophagus. A computed tomography (CT) angiography of the chest conducted after the "triple scope" revealed external compression from a double aortic arch resulting in distortion of the right-sided end of the c-shaped tracheal cartilaginous ring and causing it to bend inward along the lower tracheal lumen. Tracheomalacia was also noted at the level of the double aortic arch during the dynamic airway examination (Fig 2). Echocardiography after the CT angiography confirmed the presence of the double aortic arch with a dominant left arch and provided an evaluation of the origin points of the carotid arteries, and subclavian vessels and revealed normal biventricular function.

The Condition

A double aortic arch is the most common form of vascular ring. The double aortic arch has persistent right and left aortic arches that surround the esophagus and trachea

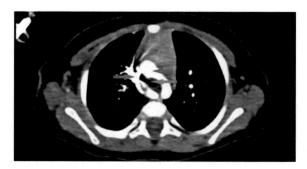

**Figure 2.** Chest CT angiography showing double aortic arch (red arrows) encircling and compressing the trachea (blue arrow). CT=computed tomography.

and cause compression. The arches then rejoin to form a common descending aorta and, as a result, completely encircle the esophagus and trachea. A double aortic arch accounts for 1% to 3% of all congenital cardiac defects. (2) As seen with our patient, the diagnosis is made via direct visualization of the airway with flexible and rigid bronchoscopy in conjunction with the thoracic imaging to evaluate the thoracic vasculature. There are also noncircumferential vascular rings that are often asymptomatic. The most common noncircumferential vascular ring is a pulmonary sling. A pulmonary sling occurs when the left pulmonary artery arises from the right pulmonary artery instead of the main pulmonary artery. This aberrant left pulmonary artery then courses between the trachea and the esophagus, creating a posterior compression of the distal trachea and anterior compression of the esophagus. It may also cause compression of the right mainstem bronchus as it crosses over it. Vascular rings can be associated with additional congenital anomalies, with reported prevalence up to 50%. (3) The majority are associated with a second cardiac lesion, but noncardiac lesions such as TEF, cleft-lip palate, and genetic and malformation syndromes such as 22q11 deletion may also be present.

## Patient Course

Our patient was referred to cardiothoracic surgery for surgical repair. The repair of a double aortic arch involves ligating the smaller of the two arches, which is usually the left arch. Ligation of the minor arch relieves the physical compression of the airway and improves the stridor. However, the consequences of long-standing compression from the vascular ring during normal cartilaginous development can be seen in the form of cartilaginous compression or stenosis of the trachea and consequent tracheomalacia. Persistent mild tracheomalacia has been seen in a small number of patients several years after repair but improves with growth over time. (4)

## Lessons for the Clinician

- Clinicians should keep a low threshold for comprehensive airway evaluation by ENT, pulmonology, and GI in young patients who have persistent stridor particularly biphasic stridor, and/or recurrent URIs.
- Close attention should be paid to the quality of the stridor on examination, along with any alleviating or aggravating factors.

*References for this article can be found at*
https://doi.org/10.1542/pir.2022-005577

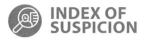

INDEX OF
SUSPICION

# Tachypnea and Epistaxis in a Full-term Infant

Daniela Titchiner, MD,* Priya Dukes, MD,* Rebecca Speier, MD,* Sharla Rent, MD*

*Duke University Hospital, Durham, NC

## CASE PRESENTATION: TACHYPNEA AND EPISTAXIS IN A FULL-TERM INFANT

A 3.8-kg male infant is born at 40 weeks' gestation to a 30-year-old primigravida woman via normal spontaneous vaginal delivery. The pregnancy is uncomplicated, with appropriate prenatal care. Delivery is uneventful; the patient receives routine delivery care with Apgar scores of 7 at 1 minute and 9 at 5 minutes. The infant is transferred to newborn nursery with no complications. At 19 postnatal hours, he develops persistent tachypnea and stertor. The patient's nares are suctioned bilaterally, followed by frank epistaxis and 2 episodes of bloody emesis. As a result, he is admitted to the NICU due to concern for respiratory distress and evaluation of bloody emesis.

Initial examination in the NICU reveals an appropriate for gestational age term infant with mild tachypnea with RR 80, no increased work of breathing, saturating > 97% on room air. Chest radiograph demonstrates no abnormalities. The results of a complete blood cell count and coagulation studies are within normal limits. The examining NICU physician notes a soft-tissue mass in the left nasal meatus, without facial asymmetry or visible oropharynx abnormality noted. Pediatric otolaryngology (ENT) department is consulted and via flexible fiberoptic laryngoscopy visualizes a "soft, pink, mass in the left nare that fluctuates with valsalva with ball-in-valve phenomenon" (Fig 1). Considering the broad differential from nasal polyp to encephalocele, neurosurgery was consulted. Magnetic resonance imaging (MRI) of the brain and computed tomography (CT) scan of facial bones show a left intranasal mass with rightward septal deviation with no definite tract diagnostic of an encephalocele (Figs 2 and 3), and the patient is scheduled for surgery with ENT for removal of mass.

## DISCUSSION

### Actual Diagnosis

Endoscopic resection of tumor is performed under general anesthesia. The tumor is polypoid in nature, broadly based along the lateral nasal wall, along the superior border of the left inferior turbinate, extending anterior to middle turbinate between the lateral nasal wall and nasal septum with right septal deviation, nearly obstructing the right nasal cavity (Fig 4). Endoscopic, gross total resection is performed. Intraoperatively, no definite intracranial connection is identified. The tissue is stained with immunohistochemical for glial fibrillary acid protein and is positive for glial tissue, consistent with diagnosis of nasal glial heterotopia.

### The Condition

Congenital nasal anomalies occur in 1 in 20,000 to 40,000 live births with 5% of them being nasal glial heterotopia or nasal gliomas with a male-to-female

AUTHOR DISCLOSURE Drs Titchiner, Dukes, Speier, and Rent have disclosed no financial relationships relevant to this article. This commentary does not contain a discussion of an unapproved/investigative use of a commercial product/device.

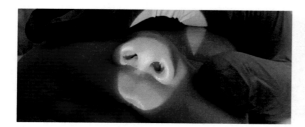

**Figure 1.** View of mass during initial physical examination.

predominance of 3:1. (1)(2) Sixty percent of these masses will be identified in the nasal subcutaneous tissue, 30% in the nasal cavity, and 10% will be a mixed presentation. (3) Overall, 10% to 15% of gliomas have a connection to the dura. (4)(5) Though not a true neoplasm, they can present similarly to other tumorlike conditions in newborns or young children. For the neonate who presents with a nasal mass, a high index of suspicion is required, despite a benign appearance.

### Differential Diagnosis

Though rare, congenital nasal masses can be a diagnostic challenge for clinicians. Categorizing congenital nasal masses into embryological origins can be helpful in broadening a clinician's differential, including ectodermal tumors

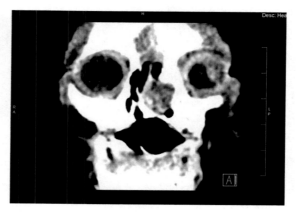

**Figure 3.** CT scan of face showing a left anterior nasal lesion with localized mass effect. No evidence of direct connection with intracranial parenchyma.

(such as dermoid), mesodermal lesions (lipomas, rhabdomyosarcomas, sinus pericranii), and neuroectodermal abnormalities (neurofibromas and basal encephaloceles). (6)(7) The differential diagnosis should also include other causes of nasal obstruction that though not congenital, can present with similar clinical symptoms. These include the following:

1. Vascular lesions, such as hemangiomas, the most common benign head and neck tumor in the pediatric population. If present on the nose they tend to grow rapidly and often show limited tendency toward involution, which can lead to signs similar to our patient; (8)

2. Choanal atresia, the most common cause of neonatal nasal obstruction, is often associated with other malformations, and is more commonly found unilaterally. If bilateral, choanal atresia can present with significant respiratory distress, which improves with crying, and an inability to pass a catheter through either nasal passages; (9) and

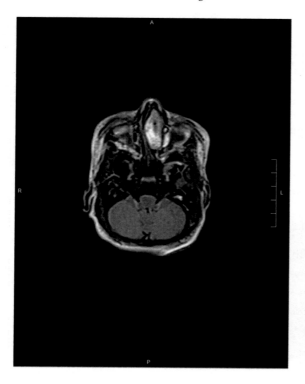

**Figure 2.** MRI of the brain showing a left intranasal mass with rightward septal deviation.

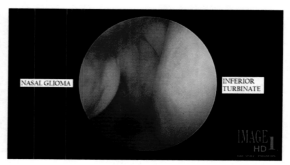

**Figure 4.** Anterior aspect of left nasal mass illustrating mobile, polypoid lesion in the anterior nare.

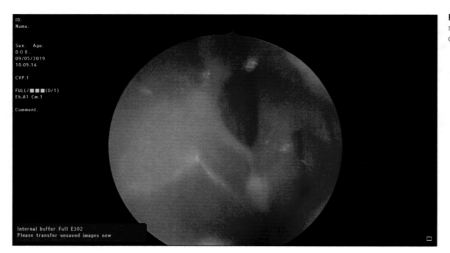

**Figure 5.** Five weeks postoperative nasal endoscopy; no clinical evidence of recurrence.

3. other nasal abnormalities such as nasal polyposis, or other noncongenital lesions.

## Management

Based upon clinical suspicion for a possible nasal glioma, the use of adjunctive imaging such as CT scans and MRIs is recommended to evaluate for a possible intracranial component or bony defect in the floor of the anterior cranial fossa, with MRI being the preferred modality for assessing the frontonasal region in the pediatric population. (10) However, even with high resolution imaging, the intracranial communication may be too small for adequate visualization, and a definitive diagnosis is often only available once surgical excision is completed. (1) Though there has been a push toward using endoscopy to aid in the evaluation of nasal masses, it presents a special challenge in pediatrics, especially in the newborn population, due to small nasal cavities and anatomical variation of landmarks. A multidisciplinary approach involving otolaryngology, neurosurgery, and neuroradiology becomes indispensable in determining the best surgical approach. (11)

## Treatment

The treatment of choice is surgical excision, with a preference toward endoscopic extracranial resection. Though these masses are benign and slow growing, if left untreated they can often lead to distortion of the nasal septum or nasal bone and can predispose the patient to infection. Overall, the recurrence rate is between 4% and 10%, requiring close follow-up and providing anticipatory guidance to parents or caretakers. (11)(12)(13)

## Patient Course

The patient was discharged from the hospital 2 days after surgical intervention with no further complications, for close follow-up by ENT and primary care providers. A 5-week postoperative nasal endoscopy showed no clinical evidence of recurrence (Fig 5).

## Lessons for the Clinician

- Nasal masses in newborns are a rare occurrence requiring clinicians to be aware of the broad differential, and a high suspicion for anomalies with intracranial extension.
- It is important that while awaiting radiographic confirmation, aspiration or instrumentation of a nasal mass should be avoided, as manipulating an encephalocele can be dangerous, and could lead to serious infections.
- Parents should be reassured that outcomes tend to be favorable, but there is a risk for recurrence. Anticipatory guidance should focus on signs of recurrence such as increase work of breathing, tachypnea, or noisy breathing.
- Due to the risk of recurrence, and thus the need for further surgical intervention, patients should be closely followed by their subspecialty physicians. (7)

## ACKNOWLEDGMENTS

Thanks to Drs Michael Cotten and Jeffrey Cheng for their review of the manuscript.

*References for this article can be found at*
https://doi.org/10.1542/pir.2022-005577

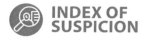

## INDEX OF SUSPICION

# Teenager with Anosmia

Caitlin L. Montgomery, MD, IBCLC,* Manisha Panchal, MD*

*Palo Alto Medical Foundation, Santa Clara Pediatrics, Santa Clara, CA

## PRESENTATION

A 16-year-old girl presents with concerns regarding the inability to smell. She has had chronic nasal congestion for the past 2 years and anosmia for the past year. She denies fever, headaches, sinus pressure, hypogeusia, or sore throat. She has regular menses. As a competitive athlete the patient has excellent activity tolerance, experiencing no cough, dyspnea, mucus production, or chest pain. She has minimal rhinorrhea in the morning, which improves throughout the day.

Her medical history reveals diagnoses of eczema, food allergies, and environmental allergies. She was diagnosed as having clinical sinusitis at age 11 years in the setting of increasingly thick nasal secretions, cough, headache, fatigue, and left-sided facial pain. She was successfully treated at that time with outpatient antibiotic drug therapy and a nasal corticosteroid and had complete resolution of her symptoms until age 16 years.

Six months ago she was seen for anosmia and nasal congestion for several months. She was diagnosed as having chronic sinusitis after a sinus culture grew heavy group B β-hemolytic streptococci. She was treated with a 14-day course of amoxicillin, a short course of prednisone, nasal corticosteroids, antihistamines, and sinus washes.

Although the previously mentioned treatments temporarily ameliorated the patient's symptoms, her anosmia and nasal congestion have recurred, prompting a return visit. Her temperature is 98°F (36.7°C) and weight is 100 lb (45.4 kg) (8th percentile). On examination she is well appearing, with left septal deviation, thick clear secretions of the left nasal passages, bilateral midturbinate hypertrophy, and 2+ tonsillar hypertrophy. There are palpable cervical lymph nodes in the anterior triangle. Her cardiorespiratory examination findings are normal. There is no hepatosplenomegaly.

Flexible nasopharyngoscopy shows polyps emerging from the left middle meatus, large polypoid tissue pushing into the right turbinate, and purulent material in the sphenoid sinus. Sinus computed tomography (CT) scan shows complete opacification of the paranasal sinuses and polypoid opacification of the nasal cavities (Fig 1).

## DISCUSSION

### Differential Diagnosis

Anosmia, defined as the inability to smell, occurs in up to 20% of the population. (1) Causes of anosmia in children may include head trauma; congenital

**AUTHOR DISCLOSURE:** Drs Montgomery and Panchal have disclosed no financial relationships relevant to this article. This commentary does not contain a discussion of an unapproved/ investigative use of a commercial product/device.

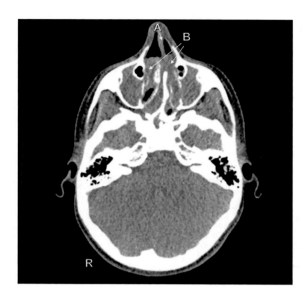

**Figure 1.** Sinus computed tomographic axial view demonstrating left nasal septal deviation (A), nasal polyps (B), and the nasal cavity and maxillary sinus with significant opacification.

olfactory disorders, which either can be isolated conditions such as idiopathic congenital anosmia (due to absence or hypoplasia of the olfactory bulbs, not associated with other congenital anomalies) or can occur as part of a multisystem condition, including Kallmann syndrome, CHARGE syndrome, 22q11 deletion (DiGeorge) syndrome, and cystic fibrosis (CF); allergic etiologies; infections, especially SARS-CoV-2 (COVID-19); toxic exposures (including smoking and pollution); nasal tumors such as juvenile nasopharyngeal angiofibromas; neurodegenerative diseases; and autoimmune diseases. (2)(3) In both pediatric and adult populations, rhinologic disease is the most common cause of decreased sense of smell. (2)(3) This may include allergic rhinitis, viral upper respiratory illness–associated anosmia, and chronic rhinosinusitis with or without polyps.

Olfaction is known to be impacted by inflammation. Up to 40% of patients with allergic rhinitis report olfactory dysfunction. (4) The ability to smell can also be impacted by coexistent anatomic abnormalities (septal deviation, turbinate hypertrophy, nasal obstruction). (2) In our patient, both factors likely play a role.

Although chronic rhinosinusitis can lead to the development of nasal polyps, most children do not go on to develop polyps. Notable exceptions include pediatric patients with CF, allergic fungal rhinosinusitis, and aspirin-exacerbated respiratory disease. (5) Patients with aspirin-exacerbated respiratory disease typically present with asthma, nasal congestion with nasal polyps, and respiratory symptoms associated with

the intake of aspirin and other nonsteroidal anti-inflammatory drugs. Our patient did not have any asthma-related symptoms. In this patient with atopy, allergic fungal rhinosinusitis should be included among the differential diagnoses; however, the clinical criteria for diagnosis of acute fungal rhinosinusitis requires the presence of fungi on culture from a mucus specimen. (6)

A thorough history may help determine the cause of anosmia. Regarding viral etiologies, anosmia and hyposmia have been frequently associated with SARS-CoV-2 (COVID-19) infection. Isolated congenital anosmia, although believed to be a rare cause of pediatric anosmia, has been implicated in up to 11% of cases in more recent literature. (2) Rare diseases, such as CF or Kallman syndrome, would be less likely differential diagnoses of anosmia and chronic rhinosinusitis because they are usually multisystem conditions.

Nasal endoscopy and imaging modalities may aid in the diagnosis and management of refractory cases of anosmia. (1) CT is helpful for evaluating traumatic and paranasal causes of anosmia, and magnetic resonance imaging can aid in diagnosing intracranial masses and evaluating the olfactory bulbs in patients with suspected idiopathic congenial anosmia. (2)

## Actual Diagnosis

Sweat chloride testing was performed and was positive at 74 mEq/L (74 mmol/L). According to the Cystic Fibrosis Foundation and the Clinical and Laboratory Standards Institute, the reference range for sweat chloride concentration is as follows: normal, less than 30 mEq/L (<30 mmol/L) (CF is unlikely); borderline, 30 to 59 mEq/L (30–59 mmol/L) (warrants further evaluation for CF); and pathological, 60 mEq/L or greater (≥60 mmol/L) (diagnostic of CF when there is appropriate clinical context). Cystic fibrosis transmembrane conductance regulator (CFTR) diagnostic gene sequencing revealed *CFTR* mutations (TG)13-5T/(TG)13-5T. The patient was diagnosed as having CF and referred to the appropriate subspecialists for ongoing management.

Interestingly, the patient was found to be pancreatic sufficient by fecal elastase and had no gastrointestinal symptoms. Initial chest CT showed minimal diffuse bronchial wall thickening and minimal air trapping of the posteromedial left lower lobe. Spirometry conveyed excellent lung function. Sputum culture revealed 3+ *Staphylococcus aureus,* for which a 21-day course of amoxicillin-clavulanate was completed. Anosmia in the setting of chronic rhinosinusitis with nasal polyposis was the primary presenting symptom of this patient's underlying CF.

Notably, the patient's newborn screening results were unattainable. Although newborn screening was first attempted in the 1970s, (7) legislation mandating universal CF testing throughout all 50 states was not in effect until 2010, (8) including the patient's birth state. Although CF is now included in the newborn screening program in all states, the method of screening and the algorithm for follow-up testing varies from state to state. Initial blood testing in every state consists of measuring the level of an infant's immunoreactive trypsinogen, a chemical produced by the pancreas, which is commonly high in patients with CF. For infants with positive newborn screening results for CF, subsequent testing regarding repeated immunoreactive trypsinogen versus DNA testing for specific CF mutations varies among states. (8)

## The Condition

CF is an autosomal recessive genetic disorder caused by the dysfunctional ion transport of sodium and chloride across epithelial cell membranes in the body. (9) This leads to the accumulation of viscous mucus that can damage several organs, which may result in progressive lung destruction, recurrent lung infections, exocrine pancreatic insufficiency, male infertility, diabetes, and malnutrition. Sinonasal disease develops in most patients with CF. The impaired mucociliary clearance and chronic inflammation of the sinonasal cavity commonly causes anosmia, headaches, rhinorrhea, and chronic nasal congestion. Our patient experienced these sinus-related symptoms of CF but has not developed any other organ involvement. This may be explained by her specific CFTR gene mutation.

CF is caused by more than 2,000 mutations in the CFTR gene. (10) Our patient's mutation, the 5T variant, refers to 5 thymidines in intron 8 of the CFTR gene, "which disrupts processing of CFTR mRNA and reduces synthesis from the corresponding CFTR alleles." (11) This well-documented polymorphism is known to have milder clinical symptoms and a variable phenotype. (11) Knowing our patient's genetic variant helps to explain her nonclassical, late-onset CF presentation.

Anosmia and hyposmia are reported in up to 71% of patients with CF. (9) Many patients with CF underestimate their smell dysfunction due to early onset of the disease in childhood. In addition, the severity of other medical issues from CF may take priority in some patients. (10) Nevertheless, patient-reported quality of life is significantly impacted by anosmia and may have serious implications regarding nutrition, which in turn impacts lung function and mortality. (12) Because our patient had a milder phenotypic presentation with later-onset CF, she was able to definitively notice when her anosmia occurred.

## Management

Management of anosmia depends on its etiology. For this patient, management of her underlying CF involves a multidisciplinary team. For upper respiratory illness–associated anosmia, most patients spontaneously recover. (1) In patients with olfactory dysfunction related to chronic rhinosinusitis, treatment includes facilitating mucociliary clearance and allowing for sinus drainage with saline irrigation. Intranasal corticosteroid sprays can help address local inflammation. For patients with signs of active bacterial infection or if symptoms are worsening/not improving, antibiotics may be beneficial. If a patient is not responding to standard first-line treatments, referral to an otolaryngologist and/or allergist may be warranted. For children with olfactory dysfunction due to allergic rhinitis, allergy testing may prove informative as patients with sinusitis have a higher incidence of positive skin prick testing. (5) Antiallergic treatments, including antihistamines, topical corticosteroids, and immunotherapy, have been shown to improve olfactory function in patients with allergic rhinitis, although data are limited. (4)

On further evaluation by an otolaryngologist, nasal polyps were detected in our patient. Nasal polyps are inflammatory growths of the sinus mucosa resulting from chronic inflammation. They occur in 20% of patients with chronic rhinosinusitis and commonly present with nasal congestion, obstruction, and anosmia or hyposmia. (13) They are known to be associated with bacterial infections, fungal infections, allergies, asthma, CF, and aspirin sensitivity. (14) Most of the literature on children with nasal polyposis is associated with CF. Between 6% and 47% of patients with CF have nasal polyps. (15) It is important for all providers to consider CF as an underlying etiology for patients presenting with nasal polyposis. As described previously herein, varying phenotypes of CF may be present, so providers should maintain a high index of suspicion, even if the patient does not fit the classical CF presentation.

Similar to the management of chronic rhinosinusitis without polyps, the treatment of nasal polyposis includes relief of sinus drainage, topical intranasal glucocorticoids, treatment of allergies, and antibiotic drug therapy. Surgical management is reserved for cases refractory to medical treatment. (14) The impact of septal deviation and septoplasty on sense of smell is unclear. A study including both adults and teenagers, found improvement in olfactory function in 70% of patients after surgery. (16) Our patient ultimately had sinus surgery for removal of her polyps and correction of her deviated septum, with subsequent improvement in her sense of smell.

## Lessons for the Clinician

- For patients with symptoms of rhinosinusitis and anosmia who do not improve on standard therapy, referral to a pediatric otorhinolaryngologist and/or allergist for further evaluation may be warranted.
- For children with nasal polyps, a sweat test should be considered, even in an older child or teenager.
- Due to phenotypic variations, some patients may have a delayed diagnosis of cystic fibrosis.

*References for this article can be found at*
https://doi.org/10.1542/pir.2021-005328.

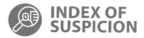

## INDEX OF SUSPICION

# The "Origin" of the Lower Lobe Opacity

Madison L. Marvel, MD,* Rasheda J. Vereen, MD, MBS,* Caitlin M. Drumm, MD,* Margaret E. Gallagher, MD*

*San Antonio Uniformed Services Health Education Consortium, San Antonio, TX

## CASE PRESENTATION

An appropriate-for–gestational age girl is born at 30 1/7 weeks' gestational age after a prenatal diagnosis of dicentric chromosome 18:22 with a 14-megabase deletion of 18q in the setting of concern for prenatal growth restriction and rocker bottom feet on ultrasonography. The mother is a 25-year-old with a history of cesarean delivery at 34 weeks for concern of uterine rupture after an intrauterine myelomeningocele repair. The prenatal course is otherwise uncomplicated, and prenatal serologies are negative. In the setting of worsening maternal abdominal pain and premature contractions, the infant is delivered emergently via cesarean delivery due to concern for maternal uterine rupture.

In the delivery room, the infant requires continuous positive airway pressure for respiratory distress and hypoxia. She is admitted to the NICU due to prematurity, where she requires escalation of respiratory support due to hypoxemic respiratory failure. She is intubated and receives surfactant on day 1 after birth. Her birth chest radiograph is significant for diffuse opacification of the bilateral lungs with air bronchograms, consistent with respiratory distress syndrome of prematurity. She remains intubated for 6 days, after which she is extubated and weaned slowly from noninvasive support. Screening imaging is completed due to her large megabase deletion and associated risk of malformations. Complete abdominal ultrasonography is normal. Echocardiogram is notable for a small, muscular ventricular septal defect. Cranial ultrasonography reveals a grade 1 germinal matrix hemorrhage on the left.

On day 52 after birth the patient requires an escalation from low-flow to high-flow nasal cannula, with chest radiography revealing a right lower lung opacity (Fig 1). Follow-up chest radiography with a lateral view shows a curvilinear opacity overlying the heart, with silhouetting of the diaphragm. On review, less apparent right lower lung opacity is seen on previous radiographs. Without further intervention, the patient's respiratory status improves with time, and she is weaned to room air on day 62 after birth.

As the patient works on oromotor skills, she is noted to have episodes of choking, concerning for aspiration. On day 67 after birth, video fluoroscopic swallow study confirms significant aspiration, likely secondary to hypotonia and discoordination associated with her underlying chromosomal deletion. Ultimately, the decision is made to place a gastrostomy tube with Nissen fundoplication. A preoperative upper gastrointestinal study is performed, the result of which is normal. The patient subsequently has a laparoscopic Nissen fundoplication and gastrostomy performed, at which point the etiology of the right lower lung opacity is discovered (Fig 2).

**AUTHOR DISCLOSURE:** Drs Marvel, Vereen, Drumm, and Gallagher have disclosed no financial relationships relevant to this article. This commentary does not contain a discussion of an unapproved/investigative use of a commercial product/device. The views expressed herein are those of the authors and do not reflect the official policy or position of Brooke Army Medical Center, the US Army Medical Department, the Defense Health Agency, the US Army Office of the Surgeon General, the Department of the Army, the Department of the Air Force, or the Department of Defense or the US Government.

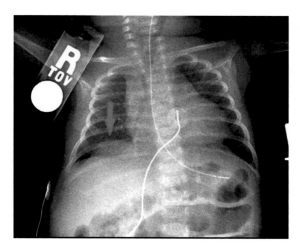

**Figure 1.** Chest radiograph obtained on day 52 after birth revealing right lower lung opacity (red arrow).

## DISCUSSION

### Differential Diagnosis

The differential diagnosis for a right lower lung opacification seen on radiography in a neonate is broad and includes diagnoses of intrapulmonary, extrapulmonary, or diaphragmatic origin. Intrapulmonary consolidations include, but are not limited to, atelectasis, pneumonia, pulmonary sequestration, congenital pulmonary airway malformation, and mass. Extrapulmonary etiologies include pleural effusion or liver mass. Diaphragmatic etiologies include diaphragmatic eventration (DE), diaphragmatic paralysis, paraesophageal hernia, and congenital diaphragmatic hernia (CDH). (1) A diaphragmatic etiology must be strongly considered in this case given the appearance of a focal elevation of the diaphragm.

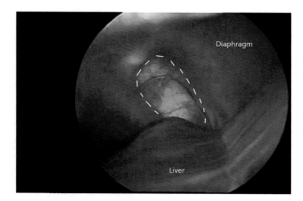

**Figure 2.** During laparoscopic surgery for the Nissen fundoplication and gastrostomy tube placement, the right diaphragm was visualized over the liver and noted to have a small defect with a hernia sac (outlined by dashed line), revealing the origin of the right lower lung opacity seen on the chest radiograph.

### Actual Diagnosis

CDHs are full-thickness defects in the diaphragm that may allow the passage of abdominal viscera into the thoracic cavity. CDH occurs in 2.4 to 3.3 per 10,000 births. (2) Forty to fifty percent of CDH cases are associated with other congenital anomalies and may be associated with a known syndrome. (1) The phenotype of 18q deletion syndrome is variable, and prognosis is based on the size and location of the deletion. In a previous study, there were no gastrointestinal or diaphragmatic anomalies linked to specific gene deletions on the long arm of chromosome 18. (3) However, 1 case series reported a patient who presented with malrotation who subsequently was found to have an 18q deletion. (4) Although we did not find any case reports of CDH associated with 18q deletion syndrome, it is well-known that CDH is associated with trisomy 18. (1)

### The Condition

Classically, CDH occurs on the left due to the lack of a solid visceral organ, the liver, preventing herniation into the thoracic cavity. In our patient, the diaphragmatic defect is on the right, which occurs in approximately 12% to 25% of cases. (5) There are different types of CDHs described by anatomic location, including posterolateral hernias (Bochdalek) and nonposterolateral hernias (Morgagni, central, and associated with pentalogy of Cantrell). Posterolateral hernias compose 80% to 90% of CDHs. (1) Classically, infants with large posterolateral defects have comorbid pulmonary hypoplasia, which presents as respiratory distress at birth requiring mechanical ventilation and occasionally extracorporeal membrane oxygenation. (6) Pulmonary hypoplasia is multifactorial, resulting from the primary defect and secondary to competition in the thoracic space. (7) Our patient required respiratory support at the time of birth, which is more likely related to respiratory distress syndrome in the setting of her prematurity.

Approximately 60% of CDHs are detected prenatally. (5) Minor defects can be missed on anatomic scans. Right-sided defects are more commonly missed due to the similar echogenicity of the liver and the lung. (1) In 1 study, 67% of right-sided CDHs were diagnosed postnatally. (5) More subtle cases may present with minor respiratory distress at birth, delayed-onset respiratory distress, chronic respiratory concerns, intestinal obstruction, and chronic gastrointestinal complaints. (8) Cases of CDHs presenting in adulthood are documented, and it is estimated that one-fourth to one-half of those are diagnosed incidentally. (9) Had our patient not required a gastrostomy tube, it is possible that her CDH would have gone undetected given her clinical improvement.

The chest radiograph in our patient was initially presumed to be consistent with DE. DEs are due to an incomplete muscularization of the diaphragm resulting in a thin membrane separating the abdominal and thoracic cavities. A small CDH can be difficult to distinguish from DE; in fact, DE and CDH can coexist. (1) Due to a thin nonmuscularized membrane there can be an elevation or bulging in the diaphragm on imaging. Some DEs can be distinguished from a CDH on radiographs alone, although more sensitive studies are ultrasonography or magnetic resonance imaging. One study used ultrasonography to look at specific criteria to distinguish CDH from DE; ultrasonography had 100% sensitivity for diagnosing CDH and only 62% specificity. The confirmatory diagnosis was made during surgical correction of the defects. (10)

DE is more common than CDH and is estimated to occur in 1 in 10,000 persons, although it is likely underdiagnosed given that many patients are asymptomatic. (11) Clinically, the bulging diaphragm and competition for thoracic cavity space can result in respiratory distress and pulmonary hypoplasia requiring respiratory support similar to CDH. (12) Some patients may present with more chronic symptoms, such as nonspecific gastrointestinal complaints. (13) Commonly, DE is not diagnosed until adulthood or is found incidentally on imaging. (14)

## Treatment

The treatment for CDHs is surgical correction, and most patients require intensive supportive care in the neonatal period. Surgery is even often completed for small asymptomatic lesions due to the risk of future bowel incarceration and obstruction. (1) Symptomatic DE may also require surgical correction through plication. (13) CDH has significant mortality associated with respiratory and gastrointestinal complications. In 1 study, it was found to have an overall mortality rate of 32.5%, but this rate significantly varies based on the severity of pulmonary hypoplasia and hypertension, the underlying etiology, and syndromic association. In the same study, when CDH was associated with a genetic syndrome, the mortality rate was noted to be as high as 82%. (15)

## Patient Course

Our patient underwent a laparoscopic Nissen fundoplication and gastrostomy. During the surgery she was noted incidentally to have a small right-sided CDH with hernia sac (Fig 2). Intraoperatively, the decision was made to defer repair given the appearance of the defect, her lack of respiratory symptoms, her stability on room air preoperatively, and her current weight and size. After her procedure, she was again weaned off respiratory support and was advanced to full enteral feeds. The CDH was then repaired at 6 months without complication.

## Lessons for the Clinician

- The most common type of congenital diaphragmatic hernia (CDH) is a left posterolateral defect.
- Sixty percent of CDHs are detected prenatally, with minor defects and right-sided defects being more commonly missed. (5)
- Diaphragmatic eventration is an incomplete muscularization of the diaphragm resulting in a thin membrane separating the abdominal and thoracic cavities; this may be difficult to distinguish from a small CDH.

*References for this article can be found at*
https://doi.org/10.1542/pir.2021-005317.

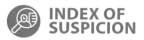

## INDEX OF SUSPICION

# Wheezing and Hypereosinophilia in a 3-year-old Girl

Smitha Hosahalli Vasanna, MD,* Peter Paul Lim, MD,† Sanjay Ahuja, MD*

*Department of Pediatrics, Division of Pediatric Hematology/Oncology,
†Department of Pediatrics, Division of Pediatric Infectious Diseases, Rainbow Babies and Children's Hospital/University Hospitals, Cleveland, OH

## PRESENTATION

A 3-year-old, unvaccinated, otherwise healthy girl presents to her clinician with a new onset of cough and wheezing that began 3 weeks ago. She has no associated fever, weight loss, rash, diarrhea, or anorexia. Her chest radiograph demonstrates opacity in the left lower lung lobe, which prompted a 10-day course of amoxicillin and a single dose of dexamethasone for presumed viral respiratory tract infection with superimposed bacterial pneumonia. With the aforementioned intervention, her symptoms improved transiently until 4 weeks later, when her parents noticed recurrence of wheezing and cough that were not associated with exertion. She is then reevaluated by her primary care physician, who diagnosed her with bilateral acute otitis medium and prescribed a second course of amoxicillin. A repeat chest radiograph did not show any opacity or abnormal finding. Owing to persistent cough with evident wheezing on physical examination in the setting of a strong family history of asthma and normal chest radiograph results, a provisional diagnosis of reactive airway disease/asthma is considered. She is initiated on levalbuterol and a 5-day course of prednisone at a dose of 1 mg/kg twice daily.

During this visit (which is 8 weeks since the onset of cough and wheezing), her parents report that she has been occasionally eating dirt. The clinician ordered blood work, which returned the next day showing a leukocytosis of $44.0 \times 10^9$/L, warranting prompt evaluation in the emergency department. There are no reports of fever, weight loss, mouth ulcers, joint pain or swelling, or known food or drug allergies or eczema. There is no report of recent travel. Her pet animals include two dogs and two pigs. She lives on a farm in northern Ohio with her parents.

She is awake, alert, and comfortable on physical examination, with a temperature of 98°F (36.66°C); heart rate, 100 beats/min; respiratory rate, 22 breaths/min; blood pressure, 98/66 mm Hg; and oxygen saturation, 98% on room air. Her weight and height are in the 81st and 85th percentiles, respectively. There is no lymphadenopathy or rash. She demonstrates intermittent expiratory wheeze on examination of her bilateral lung fields but appears comfortable. She has no rash or dry skin. Examinations of the heart, abdomen, and nervous systems are all normal. Laboratory assessment includes a white blood cell count of $52 \times 10^9$/L (reference range [RR]: $5.0–17.0 \times 10^9$/L), with absolute neutrophil count, $9.88 \times 10^9$/L (RR: $1.50–7.00 \times 10^9$/L); absolute lymphocyte count, $16.12 \times 10^9$/L (RR: $2.50–8.00 \times 10^9$/L); absolute eosinophil count, $24.96 \times 10^9$/L (RR: $0.00–0.70 \times 10^9$/L); absolute monocyte count, $1.04 \times 10^9$/L (RR: $0.10–1.40 \times 10^9$/L); hemoglobin, 12.3 g/dL (RR: 11.5–13.5 g/dL); and platelet count, $478 \times 10^9$/L (RR: $150–400 \times 10^9$/L). Erythrocyte sedimentation rate is 22 mm/h (RR: 0–13 mm/h). Her chemistries, including the

**AUTHOR DISCLOSURE:** Drs Hosahalli Vasanna, Lim, and Ahuja have disclosed no financial relationships relevant to this article. This commentary does contain a discussion of an unapproved/investigative use of a commercial product/device.

**Table 1.** Causes of HE

| HYPEREOSINOPHILIC STATES | |
| --- | --- |
| **SECONDARY/REACTIVE HE** | **DISEASE STATES** |
| 1. Infections | Parasitic (*Toxocara, Toxoplasma, Strongyloides stercoralis, Ascaris, Trichinella, Echinococcus, Microfilaria* species)<br>Fungal (*Coccidioides* species) |
| 2. Allergic (atopic and nonatopic) diseases | Asthma<br>Eczema<br>Allergic rhinitis<br>ABPA |
| 3. Medications | Antibiotics (penicillin, cephalosporins)<br>NSAIDs, antiepileptics<br>DRESS (sulfa drugs, hydantoin, hydrochlorothiazide, cyclosporine) |
| 4. Organ-restricted diseases with HE | Eosinophilic esophagitis<br>Inflammatory bowel disease<br>Cystitis<br>Pneumonia |
| 5. Autoimmune diseases | Systemic lupus erythematosus<br>Inflammatory arthritis<br>Dermatomyositis<br>Sarcoidosis |
| 6. Hematologic/immunodeficiency | Sickle cell disease<br>Wiskott-Aldrich syndrome<br>Hyper IgE syndrome/STAT3 deficiency<br>DOCK8 deficiency<br>IPEX<br>Zap70 deficiency<br>Omenn syndrome |
| 7. Oncologic | Leukemia (AML and B-ALL)<br>Lymphomas (particularly Hodgkin and T- and B-cell) |
| 8. Miscellaneous | Adrenal insufficiency<br>GVHD<br>Solid-organ transplant<br>Cholesterol embolization |
| **PRIMARY HE** | Eosinophilic leukemia |
| **FAMILIAL HE** (autosomal dominant inheritance) | Mostly benign despite HE<br>Rarely associated with endomyocardial fibrosis and peripheral neuropathy |
| **IDIOPATHIC HE** | Diagnosis of exclusion |

ABPA=allergic bronchopulmonary aspergillosis, ALL=acute lymphoid leukemia, AML=acute myeloid leukemia, DRESS=drug reaction with eosinophilia and systemic symptoms, DOCK8=dedicator of cytokinesis 8, GVHD=graft versus host disease, HE=hypereosinophilia, Ig=immunoglobulin, IPEX=immune dysregulation, polyendocrinopathy, enteropathy, X-linked syndrome, NSAIDS=nonsteroidal anti-inflammatory drugs, STAT3=signal transducer and activator of transcription 3.

following, are all in the normal RRs: sodium, potassium, chloride, bicarbonate, blood urea nitrogen, creatinine, calcium, phosphorus, total and conjugated bilirubin, alanine aminotransferase, aspartate aminotransferase, and alkaline phosphatase. Albumin is 4.2 g/dL (RR: 3.2–4.7 g/dL), and total protein is 7.4 g/dL (RR: 5.9–7.2 g/dL). Serum immune globulin profile shows immunoglobulin (Ig) E concentration of 4,922 IU/mL (RR: 0–199 IU/mL); IgG, 999 mg/dL (RR: 335–975 mg/dL); IgA, 123 mg/dL (RR: 17–70 mg/dL); and IgM, 316 mg/dL (RR: 22–124 mg/dL).

## DISCUSSION

### Differential Diagnosis

With an absolute eosinophil count of $24.96 \times 10^9$/L, the patient has severe hypereosinophilia (HE). HE is classified as mild when the absolute eosinophil count (AEC) in the peripheral blood is greater than the upper limit of normal and $1.5 \times 10^9$/L; moderate when the AEC is between $1.5 \times 10^9$/L and $5 \times 10^9$/L cells/µL; and severe when the AEC is greater than $5 \times 10^9$/L cells/microliter. (1)(2)

Eosinophilia is usually an incidental finding in complete blood cell counts done on routine surveillance tests or as part of an evaluation for another symptom complex. The differential diagnosis for HE in children is broad and is depicted in the Table 1.

### Diagnosis and Management

The patient had multiple potential overlapping causes for HE, which include recently diagnosed presumed reactive airway disease/asthma in the setting of strong family history of atopic disorders, recent use of amoxicillin (the antibiotic most commonly described with drug-induced eosinophilia), and a history of pica, raising suspicion for a parasitic infection.

This scenario, ie, having multiple HE risk factors, is common. The patient's demographics, past and family history, concomitant symptoms, duration of eosinophilia, and, to some extent, the degree of eosinophilia are some indicators that could help narrow the differential diagnosis. Although asthma or an allergic phenomenon can cause HE, asthma is usually associated with only mild or moderate HE, and such severe HE in the setting of atopic disorders is usually associated with eczema, which the patient did not demonstrate. Antibiotics including amoxicillin have been commonly implicated in drug-induced HE. The most common presentation of drug-induced HE is a cutaneous rash; however, organ-specific toxicities such as immune-mediated hepatitis, nephritis, pneumonitis, and drug rash eosinophilia and systemic symptoms (DRESS) are described. The patient did not demonstrate any rashes or organ toxicities, although isolated drug-induced HE cannot be completely excluded. Risk factors for parasitic infections in the patient included living on a farm in the rural United States, exposure to dogs and pigs, and a history of pica. Furthermore, given her recent wheezing (pulmonary involvement) in the setting of pica and severe HE, parasitosis was high on the differential diagnosis list. Eosinophilic leukemia is characterized by the uncontrolled proliferation of eosinophilic precursors in the bone marrow with normal serum IgE concentrations. High IgE concentrations indicate cytokine (interleukin [IL]-5)-mediated reactive, also known as secondary, HE. Eosinophilia can cause tissue damage through variable mechanisms that can include infiltration, fibrosis, thrombosis, or allergic inflammation. (3)

Initial consolidation on the patient's chest radiograph could have been due to a superimposed bacterial pneumonia; her subsequent chest radiograph was normal. In pulmonary visceral larva migrans, chest radiographs are typically normal and only rarely reveal solitary nodules, whereas a computed tomography chest scan may reveal multifocal subpleural nodules with halo or ground-glass opacities. Owing to the severe degree of her eosinophilia, which implicated high potential for end-organ damage, urgent additional evaluation, including echocardiography, chest imaging, and ocular examination, were emphasized. The need for bone marrow evaluation for diagnosis if the initial evaluation was unrevealing was also discussed. Her parents declined admission and inpatient testing because she was relatively well-appearing, and outpatient evaluation ensued.

## Actual Diagnosis

Stool ova and parasitic tests, as well as giardia and cryptosporidium antigens, yielded negative results. Serological tests for strongyloidiasis and *Toxocara* species were sent to a reference laboratory, which yielded a positive-result *Toxocara canis* enzyme-linked immunosorbent assay (ELISA) and a negative-result strongyloidiasis test. To reduce cross-reactivity with antigens of *Ascaris* species and other parasites, this ELISA used the excretory-secretory antigen of *T canis* larvae. A final diagnosis of visceral larva migrans was made. Allergic bronchopulmonary aspergillosis was excluded with negative-result aspergillus antibodies by complement fixation and immunodiffusion techniques.

## The Condition

Parasites that migrate to end-organ tissues such as *Toxocara*, *Strongyloides stercoralis*, *Ascaris*, *Trichinella spiralis*, *Schistosoma*, and *Filaria* species cause notable eosinophilia. Parasitic infections that present with pulmonary symptoms and eosinophilia include toxocariasis, ascariasis, and strongyloidiasis.

Toxocariasis is caused by the larvae of the roundworm *Toxocara canis* (dog) and *Toxocara cati* (cat). Infected dogs and cats excrete *Toxocara* eggs into the environment through their feces. *Toxocara* larvae take 2 to 4 weeks of incubation within the egg to become infectious, and they can remain infectious for months to years under optimal environmental circumstances. (4) In most cases, humans become infected after ingesting dirt containing *Toxocara* eggs and, in rare cases, after consuming undercooked/raw contaminated lamb or rabbit meat. *Toxocara* species seroprevalence in the United States is reported to be 14% in earlier studies, although a recent study estimated it to be 5%. (5)(6) Ocular and visceral toxocariasis are the two main types of toxocariasis. Visceral toxocariasis or visceral larva migrans primarily affect the liver and lungs and can manifest as fever, anorexia, hepatitis, pneumonitis, pruritic urticaria, and eosinophilia. Because the adult stage of *Toxocara* species does not occur in humans, no eggs or larvae are identified in stool samples. Larval forms can only be detected in the stool of definitive hosts such as dogs and cats. Toxocariasis is diagnosed in humans using conventional methods such as blood tests (blood cell count and eosinophilia); serological tests for larval stage antigens such as excretory/secretory antigens (ELISA and Western blot); histopathological examination (to detect larvae); and/or molecular techniques such as polymerase chain reaction to detect larval DNA in tissue or body fluid samples. Treatment mainly consists of albendazole or mebendazole for 5 days.

*Strongyloides stercoralis* species is a parasite that has a similar clinical appearance but is treated differently. Humans, primates, and domestic dogs are the definitive hosts for

## Eosinophil Trend

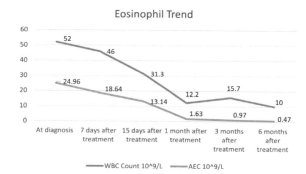

**Figure 1.** Trend in WBC count and AEC. AEC=absolute eosinophil count; WBC=white blood cell.

*Strongyloides stercoralis.* Strongyloidiasis is diagnosed by examining larvae under a microscope on a stool sample. It can be also diagnosed on biopsy specimens, in sputum, and by serological tests.

*Ascaris* infections in humans are typically caused by *Ascaris lumbricoides* (human roundworm); however, infection with *Ascaris suum* (pig roundworm) is becoming more common because of community pig farming. Based on egg morphology in stool studies, it is difficult to discriminate between *A lumbricoides* and *A suum.* However, specific ELISA-based tests are currently available that can distinguish between *Toxocara* and *Ascaris* species.

## Patient Course

The patient received a course of albendazole at 400 mg twice daily for 5 days. One week after therapy, her eosinophil count had dropped dramatically and continued to improve on subsequent blood cell counts, as depicted in the Figure 1. The patient was not receiving oral or inhaled steroids, which could otherwise be a contributory factor for the drop in the eosinophil count. Her mother also reported that her wheezing resolved and that her appetite improved after therapy. Their dogs were not tested because the family declined.

## Lessons for the Clinician

- Although parasitic infections are uncommon in the developed world, the diagnosis should be considered in the presence of risk factors.
- Toxocariasis should be in the differential diagnosis for a patient who presents with hypereosinophilia and wheezing.
- Visceral larva migrans results from migration of *Toxocara* species to the lungs of an infected patient causing pulmonary symptoms such as wheezing.
- Preferred treatment for visceral larva migrans is a 5-day course of albendazole.
- Hypereosinophilia and other associated symptoms such as wheezing improve with adequate treatment of toxocariasis.

*References for this article can be found at*
https://doi.org/10.1542/pir.2022-005728